Black Bag Moon

Doctors' Tales from Dusk to Dawn

SUSAN WOLDENBERG BUTLER

Foreword by

ALEC LOGAN

Radcliffe Publishing
London • New York

Radcliffe Publishing Ltd
33–41 Dallington Street
London
EC1V 0BB
United Kingdom

www.radcliffepublishing.com

British Library Cataloguing in Publication Data

A catalogue record for this book is available from the British Library.

ISBN-13: 978 184619 970 7

The paper used for the text pages of this book is FSC® certified. FSC (The Forest Stewardship Council®) is an international network to promote responsible management of the world's forests.

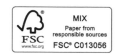

Typeset by Darkriver Design, Auckland, New Zealand
Printed and bound by TJI Digital, Padstow, Cornwall, UK

Contents

Foreword

A recent Monday morning surgery at Wishaw Health Centre, Lanarkshire, Scotland, my stomping ground.

'I have a rash,' said my first patient, a 30-something teacher. And she had: anterior chest wall, patchy itchy red rings, 3–4 centimetres in diameter. The diagnosis was obvious: a fungal infection, tinea corporis, popularly known as ringworm. Nothing to do with worms – 'ringworm' on account of appearance, not cause. I love diagnosing ringworm. It's easy to spot, treatment is simple and invariably effective.

'This is . . .' I began, then paused. I remembered an earlier consultation, over 20 years previously, in our branch surgery some miles away in Law village. Another case of ringworm, this time a young girl, with her anxious mum. 'That's ringworm!' I pronounced, with insufficiently disguised relish. And my poor young patient burst into tears. A lesson learned.

Back to the present.

'This is,' I began again, 'a fungal infection. A bit like athlete's foot. Sometimes we call it ringworm. Nothing to do with worms, of course. It's the ring-like appearance. But I've always been wary of calling it ringworm since I upset a patient many years ago . . .'

'That was me,' said my patient.

An epiphany. I had hoped for 20 years to see that girl again. I was able to apologise for my gaucheness, to tell her how much I'd learnt from my mistake, to recount how many times I'd recounted the story while teaching medical students and trainee GPs. We shook hands warmly and off she went with her prescription.

Such a classical general practice encounter. The timescale, the intimacy, the importance of small things, the glory of personal generalist doctoring.

Black Bag Moon is full of such stories. Fictionalised, anonymised, but in essence true.

Enjoy. Reflect. Demand decent family medicine!

Alec Logan
General Practitioner
Lanarkshire, Scotland
Deputy Editor, *British Journal of General Practice*
March 2012

Preface

There are some wonderful physician-writers out there. Currently, I'm reading James Willis' *The Paradox of Progress*, the late Cecil Helman and the prolific mid-twentieth-century George Sava, whose old Penguin autobiography, *The Healing Knife*, I discovered in my husband's medical library. All speak passionately and compassionately about the human condition, that never-endingly fascinating topic. How fortunate are/were their patients!

But what about the legions of general practitioners, those foot soldiers marching through the night, who haven't the time or inclination to make their voices heard? This book peeks into their lives. From air currents drifting through dinner parties and awards ceremonies, conference meals and personal interviews, I have plucked the floating petals that comprise this bouquet. For a doctor's wife who keeps her ears open, one sentence mumbled into the salad can be enough, like 'I had to put down this old miner's dog last week and I thought, how hard can it be?' This led to the second story in the chapter entitled, 'Putting Down Pooch.'

Speaking of names, you may be wondering about 'Black Bag Moon.' I had enough material for another book after completing *Secrets from the Black Bag* and wanted to explore topical issues such as HIV/AIDS, femocracy and euthanasia. I was googling Sava's book titles and found *Cocaine for Breakfast* and *They Come by Appointment*, which led me to choose one for the present work – by the seaside with scarlet-and-turquoise rosellas tweeting just outside – that had a bit of colour and magic. I hope you agree.

These stories have been created with love for those who traverse the dark angst and chaos with their patients and listen to daily recitations of sniffles and funny turns – and who bear what Dr Willis defines as, referring to weekends on call, 'The almost physical burden of waiting for things that might have happened but didn't' (p. 27). Some doctors in these pages will be familiar from *Secrets from the Black Bag*. Catch up with Tommy MacDonald, Amaranth Fillet and Dexter Veriform. Others drop in for the first time. Meet Barker Kaye, Malcolm Phillips, David Snow, Petra Neumann, Nicky Doulton-Brown and Amaranth's husband Wayne Cooperfield.

Managing my husband's medical practice in a small country town for several years before he slid completely into academia exposed other facets of the gem of general practice, if I may change metaphors, like processing patients who saved their best behaviour for Doctor, like interviewing locums who lectured on which item numbers to use to defraud the system, like welcoming such patients as the sweet Catholic nun who always smelled of roses. The gem sparkles generously as it dances towards extinction. A poem comes to mind from Tsangyang Gyatso, the rebel sixth Dalai Lama (1685–1706), miracle maker and poet of the people:

When the gem was mine
I cared not, and ignored its value.
Now that the gem is lost to others
Melancholy overwhelms me
As its pure worth dawns on me.

Susan Woldenberg Butler
Canberra
March 2012

About the author

Susan Woldenberg Butler is a freelance writer, researcher, editor and president of the Benevolent Organisation for Development, Health & Insight (BODHI). She lives with her husband, Colin, mostly in Canberra, Australia. She is the author of a previous work of medical fiction, *Secrets from the Black Bag*, and is working on a third volume.

www.susanbutler.com.au

www.bodhi.net.au

Acknowledgements

Let's rotate the gem, the world, the moon, and see what sparkles and glints.

My father was a passionate believer in the equality of all. He stood his ground when the Ku Klux Klan came to visit our home one day in 1950s Mississippi. The reason? Dad waited in the house of his black employee one morning while the latter got ready for work. My mother, to whom this book is dedicated, is a survivor, sense of black humour intact and thriving despite training at a girls' school which has been educating young ladies since the early 1800s.

The doctors whose stories are told herein cannot be named and thanked personally due to the promise of anonymity. Other *ities* spring to mind: generosity, perspicacity, personality. Some *ations* join them: inspiration, perspiration, dedication. Three *lesses* close the circle: fearless, timeless, peerless. Here comes another *ation* known for its *ities*: previous generations of medicos such as *The Fabulous Flemings of Kathmandu* (Christianity), Axel Munthe in San Michele (exclusivity) and Sir Wilfred Grenfell with the deep-sea fishermen of Labrador (physicality).

Alec Logan has added dazzle with a Foreword from his lair in Scotland. Reader Ann Bliss in Southern California and friend Pamela Hewitt in Sydney, Australia, proffered advice with panache. Agent Pat (Poland) Haarhaus, a Cherokee Indian near Cut and Shoot, Texas, is neverendingly supportive. Friend Adrian Sleigh generously answered medical questions.

Production of this book has been a global effort. Gillian Nineham at Radcliffe in England worked gleamingly to ensure that *Black Bag Moon: Doctors' Tales from Dusk to Dawn* saw the light of day. The publishing process was seamless thanks to Jamie Etherington, transplanted from England to Victoria, Australia, and Camille Lowe and her team in New Zealand. Radcliffe's marketing/publicity department has been right on the money.

Some authors accompany one on every twist of the medical literary journey: Anton Chekhov, Franz Kafka, Hervey Cleckley, William Carlos Williams, AJ Cronin, John Berger, W Somerset Maugham and André Soubiran, to name a few of many. And always, James Herriot.

The ever-(r)evolving medical humanities – with its field of stars and villains, outré and conventional, pretentious and piercing – is burning craters and making moons shine.

Last and forever, deepest gratitude to my husband, Colin, for making it all possible, wherever we find ourselves, in whatever incarnation.

Dedication

To my mother, Irene Violet Meyer Woldenberg Atles Moran . . .

Black bag moon

Barker Kaye

Aside from the bulldozer, not a human sound out here disturbs the timeless peace within cooee. No telephones ring or computers whir. My mobile phone is switched off. No radio disgorges bad news. An Emmylou Harris tape, now that's different. This song reminds me of the old standard, 'Night and Day', and of Mr Pym. Medical practice night and day. Children crying, oldies coughing, drug reps chatting and wives complaining . . . stacks of uncompleted medical reports from a mine foray . . . all the day detritus versus nocturnal drugs and sex. Femocrats come and go. Spouses come and go. Patients come and go. *We* come and go. Mr Pym remains, an urban nightmare invading the rural heart, exemplifying isolation and my inability to respond to a patient's *cri de coeur.*

It was a real black bag moon, round and beaming pale blue rays into every corner of the night, a frenetic lighthouse illuminating the peaks and troughs to creatures of the dark like myself. The black bag moon heralded the sort of night I dreaded at the after-hours medical service. One extreme or the other: constant callouts or a single life-altering experience. Which would it be tonight?

Doing locums increased my feeling of isolation. I hadn't found my niche or my bolthole despite hospital work and gigs for old friends whose eyes spoke of the settling influence of women. I didn't envy worker bees at desks, lashed ever onward by family photographs lovingly positioned on desks and children's coloured-paper paintings taped to walls. The former were framed, trapped, the latter unbordered by convention. I hated hospital politics. The trivial nature of most complaints in suburban general practice bored me. Perhaps I'd forsake medicine, work part-time or become a woodworker. Or all three. Or become a specialist: pity to waste the training. Dermatologists and urologists didn't have many home visits. Nothing appealed to me. I retained my original motivation to help – what in Buddhism is called *bodhicitta*. I watched from an ever-increasing distance as classmates slotted into definite career paths. I slipped into night work at the after-hours service to free my days for non-medical pursuits. Patients would be less predictable, less flattened into bloodless squares by life's silver bullets.

The black bag moon taught me a lot. A silent legion of us wandered the edges of the collective consciousness. Young doctors weren't the only ones to feel quarantined. Patients experienced all sorts of isolation. People rattle on about rural isolation, but in my experience urban patients bump along the bottom with the best of them, especially in the middle of the night.

People like Allan Pym.

I was working one night at the clinic during the winter after my pilgrimage to South India to earn money for my impending marriage. Around midnight, I gazed upon my urban domain, snug in an armchair I had dragged to the bay window. This Victorian parlour was now the reception room. I loved the stillness before a snowfall. I'd returned not long before from attending a sick child. Rather than attempting to sleep straight away, I needed to decompress in the dark, staring at icy streetscapes glinting in the chain of streetlights. It gave me perspective after middle-of-the-night callouts. I settled into the welcoming armchair as floating snow obscured the moon and whipped into flurries.

My wish for a peaceful night was not to be fulfilled. Ninety seconds later, the telephone blasted through the darkness.

'Dr Kaye here.'

A male voice whispered, 'Doctor, I'm HIV-positive and I want to kill myself.'

I sat upright. The streetscape lost its appeal as my focus narrowed. 'What's your name?' My hand flopped reflexively on a nearby table for a pen and chartreuse notepad advertising a new wonder drug.

'Allan Pym.'

'Well, Mr Pym, don't do anything until I arrive. What's your address?'

I was soon on the way. In my haste, I tangled my shirt and jumper. As I bent into the car, snow scalpelled across the small of my back. I jabbed at the dashboard, willing the heater to rejuvenate. No luck. I thumped the steering wheel.

Mr Pym forgot to leave a light on, so finding him took some time. My fingers were numb when I arrived at his flat. I finally parked and started for the front door. My doctor's bag slipped and I dropped it in the slushy gutter. Not a buzzer or bell in sight, so I banged at the freezing entrance with a balled fist.

A balding, thirtyish man in a purple-and-gold bathrobe opened the door. 'Come in, Dr Kaye,' he said, brushing my thigh as he closed the door behind me. He led me into the lounge, to a sofa in front of an electric fire set into a fireplace.

'Are you in the theatre?' I fished for an interest to restore to the poor man his grip on life.

Masks of different colours and ethnological backgrounds obscured the walls. The wide bulging eyes of one carved wooden head leered in a particularly terrifying way. The nostrils above its massive jaw looked like twin tunnels to hell.

Mr Pym noticed my glazed horror and smiled – obviously a great effort. 'That's a mask for a lion's dance, given to me by a shaman in Okinawa.'

'Let's sit down, Mr Pym, and perhaps you can tell me what's troubling you.'

He touched my leg as he lowered himself on the sofa, uncomfortably close.

'Mr Pym.'

'Allan, please.'

'Allan, what's troubling you?'

I looked away. His head was framed by the lion mask's wild and copious mane, cloaking him in a fierceness that made concentration difficult. I gazed into one possible future. Would I end up like this night owl, desolate at the end of the road?

'I'm lonely, Dr Kaye. May I call you . . .?' he left the question hanging.

'Dr Kaye.'

He placed his arm along the top of the sofa, near my shoulder.

'Mr Pym,' I said, moving away.

'Allan.'

'Allan, you said on the phone you were HIV-positive?'

'Yes.'

'When did you find out?'

'A few months ago.'

'Do you have anyone you can turn to?'

'No doc, I'm all alone.' Mr Pym leaned forward. 'That's why I rang you.' His purple-and-gold bathrobe fell open, revealing a fully erect penis.

I jumped up. 'Don't you ever abuse the doctor–patient relationship like that again!' I slammed the door on my way out of the house and slipped in the slush of the gutter. On my backside, I realised I'd forgotten to charge him.

Mr Pym rang the next day to apologise. He didn't settle his account and the after-hours service didn't pursue it, so I was not paid; indeed, I was never paid for subsequent telephone consultations or to comfort Mr Pym. I counselled him through the receiver about the Buddha's teachings of illness, suffering and death, but I'm afraid I was rather perfunctory and got rid of him as soon as I could. I'm not perfect. I can't always disentangle a *cri de coeur* from my emotional responses, as with Mr Pym. Nor can I always unravel my need for space from my medical vows.

Get on with it

David Snow

A rough go on 100K a year, the national average. Not bad for unskilled labour. The work's dirty and can be dangerous. The prevailing mentality round here is to chuck it and go back on the dole. They get sick of it. They don't have a saving mentality, which can be a problem when they buy a house and bring out their families. Big mortgages.

Get on with it: that's the motto of our remote community. Even with accidents. Especially with accidents. Mishaps with children have been my worst callouts. It's awful when children die, and worse when it's because of parental negligence. The saddest one I've ever attended was a two-year-old little boy who drowned in the local creek. The parents, Kevin and Katrina Simpson, were nearby but distracted by marriage turmoil. Kevin was unemployed. When miners' families have a rough go, I remind them of our motto: get on with it.

A lot of contract work's going round the country, which is disruptive to families. You come in and work in a mining camp and go home on your days off. Nobody emphasises setting up a town, which is obviously a far better arrangement: more services, like a local GP, and fewer broken marriages, but it's costly and the mining companies aren't prepared to do it. They view themselves as a business, not a service organisation, and say that we've got to get used to the idea that we're a town with mining in it, not a mining town. You know that sort of glib talk. Well no, we don't have to get used to their way of evading social responsibilities.

The biggest health problem in the rural sector is unemployment one, unemployment two, unemployment three, unemployment four and all the rest follows. Yes, it's easier to find mining work in remote areas now because mineral prices are great, but there's always job uncertainty. How do you plan for the future or take out a huge mortgage on your house when they can sack you at any time? It's pretty stressful.

Little Jayde Simpson's family knew all about that. Kev had lost his job 6 months before. It wasn't his fault. Same old story: lay-offs, and he took to the grog.

Marriage breakdown: I see a lot of that. Mining's absolutely toxic for marriages, and why not? Katrina came to see me last year, when Kev was still working. She was dead lonely, bored, caring for the kids. Kevin was either down below or chilling out on his days off. Things were improving after we got rid of the extended shift roster 9 months ago. Now it's only 4 or 5 days on, not 7 like in the past. They'd recover the first day and spend 1 or 2 days' quality time with the family, which wasn't usually at weekends when the kids were at home. Then they'd go down and do the same thing. Now the young couple had plenty of time together, which was driving them both nuts.

The day their baby died, Kevin and Katrina were having one of those awful domestics that couples do. It was just before lunch. I planned to catch up with the medical literature – well, not catch up, I'd never fully do that. Make a dent. It was a warm Tuesday in spring, which doesn't happen often, so when it does, somebody's usually down by the creek. Things might have turned out differently at a weekend or later in the day. More people would have been around and some-body might have saved Jayde. Conan, the Simpsons' older son – 5 years on this earth and uncontrollable, surprise surprise – ran off when they started arguing, Katrina told me later. They started arguing about the elder boy but soon moved on, in the manner of spousal quarrels.

I could picture it: meandering creek, bare mountain topped with snow domi-nating the town, park grounds rocky, colours changing from winter monochrome to spring green. Three wooden picnic tables and benches splattered with bird droppings and a litter bin nearby with junk-food wrappers blown against the base of its metal pole by the ever-present wind. Hungry ravens swooped with fierce curved beaks and black eyes. Native shrubs obscured the creek's bend. The park the community fought so hard for has a menacing feel. Nothing comes easily here. We just get on with it.

In my mind's eye, I watched a young family tumble out of the car and move in stages towards the tables like a mutant, spreading amoeba. Another reason to grumble: an expensive vehicle impractical for little ones. Lots of door slamming, righteous stomping and menacing facial expressions. 'I work so hard. Why can't I have me bit o' pleasure?' 'What about your family?'

Admonitions of 'Watch your brother!' were carried away by the wind and unheard by five-year-old ears. A dented blue-and-white cooler protected the food against ravens and, most important, kept the beer chilled. All wore jeans and T-shirts except Mum, who was wearing the pink tracksuit she always donned in early pregnancy. Another reason to cross swords.

A whirly-whirly – that spiralling wind that collects dust and refuse – blurred the white-bread sandwiches and black curved bird beaks, the bags of crisps and bottles of cordial. And the beer. And the hair. Katrina and Jayde were white blondes. Hers hadn't faded despite 20 years of doing it hard. His never would, now. Kev and Conan were cut from the same cloth – trouble later – both as pig-headed as the day is long, with wispy brown curls atop their stubborn heads. That mum's resentment was about to boil over showed in the way she slid Kev his sandwich. It snagged on a splinter and the plastic wrap unravelled. A typical family having some quality time.

'Watch your brother!' She went after the five-year-old. 'I'm talkin' to you –'

Sound of bottle opening. 'Leave 'im alone. You're always naggin' 'im. Like me.'

That's all it took. Both sons scattered to avoid the slanging match they knew was coming.

My mind's eye hooded itself. I knew these domestics too well, both my own and those of my patients. I dragged the eye open to confront the sight that haunts me, even though the little lad was on land when I tried to resuscitate him: poor Jayde's white-blonde hair skimming the water. Katrina hadn't even cut it, ever. He sank to his watery grave carrying every last strand he'd been born with, tangled with the weeds that claimed him. This whorled me into a reverie about the traps life sets.

Jayde's brother found him floating in the water, coated with algae and vegetation. He stepped straight into oblivion, simply walked in and sank, as a child would at that age. Kev and Conan fished him out and tried to resuscitate him with mouth-to-mouth and CPR.

Now my inner vision and reality converged. The elder son rang the surgery on Kev's mobile phone. Barely understood his shrieks. I ran straight out, yelling at the receptionist to call the ambulance. When I arrived at the creek, Ken and Conan practically carried me from the gravel parking strip to Jayde. Their clothes dripped slime. Mum's hair mingled with that of her lost baby as she held and rocked and moaned. The poor child was well and truly gone. I intubated Jayde, going through the motions, but it was pointless. Too late, too late.

Father comforted remaining son 10 feet away. Their wispy curls were matted on their scalps. 'Why did this happen to me?' 'Us, son, us.'

Mum was lost in her grief, alternately screaming 'I told you to watch him!' and burying her face in her sodden son's hair.

I couldn't say anything, so I left.

Before long, Katrina had a miscarriage. Kev disappeared with another woman 2 years after little Jayde drowned and started a new family in another town. Conan stayed on with his mum. Father and son didn't long remain in their pod, two peas united against the wife and mother who grew to hate them both. Kev's new family had no room for Conan. He symbolised the bad old days that Kev wanted to forget. Conan didn't fit into Katrina's life either. Her new partner disliked him and kept Katrina occupied with plenty of babies. The eldest boy reminded her of that awful day in the park and the bad times that followed. Nobody wanted Conan, and he knew it.

The years passed. The bigger Conan grew, the wider was the rift with his father, who found steady work in a copper mine 120 kilometres away. Problem was, Conan hated going underground. He didn't want to be like the old man. He wanted to work with computers, which scandalised his father. It was sissy.

Conan came in occasionally for the usual childhood ailments. The other day, I came across his notes in the surgery and found I'd scrawled 'SUW' consistently over the years: my shorthand for a sullen, uncommunicative and whining child. I urged him to join our football club. He wasn't very tall, but he was solid as a rock, nuggety like his father. He wasn't interested in being brought out of himself. I'd no time to counsel him after Jayde drowned, and the town lacked a psychologist. We were rough and ready, as isolated spots are. We just got on with it.

Miners spent very little on their houses because the company owned them. They waited for the company to fix them up and often waited a very long time. Cars were another story. They loved their cars and poured the dollars into them. So did their sons. Sometimes it was the only way they related, like Conan and Kev.

By the time Conan was old enough to drive, the only bond the Simpson males retained was a love for cars. As the annual automobile show approached, Conan stayed with his father every weekend. Sometimes he'd come back happy, smelling of oil and grease and rubber, and other times ready to kill, Katrina said when she brought in one baby daughter or another.

And now to the time of Conan's car accident. One night 12 years after Jayde died, Katrina produced another baby boy after a string of daughters. Kev sired only girls, three of them, with his new partner. And all the previous children of both partners were girls. That left Conan as the only son and eldest child of what Kev called a brood of hens. The latest birth was another way for father and son to be close, which they both grabbed. Kev bought a slightly used car from one of the miners and gave it to his 17-year-old son. I'd never seen Conan so happy. Perhaps this would extricate him from his personal hell pit and propel him into a new life in the city in computers.

Conan did burnouts in the street for a while, until the local policeman threatened to take away his licence. Other than that, he was conscientious with the car, considering the grim statistics of cars and teenaged boys. Until one night, a night none of us will ever forget.

Conan found himself a girlfriend, the lovely 15-year-old Nicole. She was a town girl, reared by a mother and injured father who'd been paid out by the mine and now ran a motor repair business from a small shop off the high street. Nicole helped out in the hospital and planned to be a nurse. She'd have been magnificent, and we needed her. Conan enrolled in a computer course and was starting work at the petrol station nearest his house on Monday, to save up for his living expenses. He wanted to supplement the government's living allowance, which wasn't enough to support both Conan and his car. He planned to work for a year, live at home and save his earnings, except for petrol. That was the plan, Katrina told me when she brought in her infant son for a baby check. She exhibited relief, not pride. When questioned, she whispered that she was glad. She needed his room but was sorry to see him go because he was useful round the place, if you approached him right.

Conan took Nicole out to celebrate on a spring Saturday evening with summer in the air. Temperatures still plummeted at night, turning the roads slick and icy, as was to happen in a few short hours. For now, though, life was ace for the adolescent. The town's teenagers were in that happy, end-of-school-year state. I was amazed that this problem child – the one we always love the best – finally came good despite dire predictions.

Half past eleven, the phone rang. Car accident. God I hate those calls. The ambulance picked me up and we zoomed down the main street to a windy bit of road 10 kilometres out of town. We all dread it: black as Hades outside, except for where the headlights cut through, adrenalin pumping from zero to full tilt, home life receding fast. What exactly could we expect? Scratches? Hysteria? Carnage? Unlike some doctors I knew, I trusted my abilities. I could cope with whatever came along that required my technical skills. Conan was about to add another nightmare to the collection.

We passed no other vehicles of any kind on the road. The ambulance rounded that last corner, flashing like a demented lighthouse. One pulse revealed Conan's automotive pride and joy by the roadside. He sprawled on the bonnet, staring.

He slithered off as soon as he saw me. A light speared Nicole lying on the road-side, motionless.

He ran at me. 'I haven't moved her! I haven't touched her!' he cried, blocking my way.

I shoved him aside and knelt by the girl. I picked up her head. It had the consistency of a squashed coconut: hard but soft underneath. It was terrible, terrible. It was smashed, with the skin attached.

'She wasn't wearing a seat belt! She went out head first!'

Nicole was alive when we reached her, body broken, blood pressure down, bleeding profusely. Air hunger made her gasp for breath, trying to oxygenate what little blood remained. I put in an IV line and gave her what blood we had.

I don't remember the drive to the hospital, nor do I know how Conan got there. I recall glaring overhead lights as I focused on saving the dying girl. What should I do? Keep her alive to be an organ donor? She died within half an hour. Once they've died like that, you can forget salvaging body parts.

Conan kept up a horrible chorus the entire time. He lay on the waiting-room floor, moaning, in an extreme anxiety state. We heard him hollering, 'Why me?' Took me right back to the spring day little Jayde drowned in the river.

Nicole's face was swelling up from all the oedema. We covered her head and made the body reasonable for the parents to view their daughter. They'd only been told about their daughter's involvement in a serious accident. Nothing more. I hurried to the waiting room.

I stepped over Conan and approached the nervous couple huddled together at the edge of the room. The young Simpson idiot was hyperventilating. I said to one of the sisters through gritted teeth, 'Get . . . him . . . out . . . of . . . here . . .'

Time to inform the parents. 'Come with me,' I said, leading them away. Nicole's father limped badly from his mining accident. I stopped outside the room where the poor girl lay. 'Look, I'm sorry she's gone.' I should have dragged it out and said, 'Look, I'm sorry, I'm very sorry, but she's gone.' I couldn't. God it was awful. I get teary-eyed when I think of it. They were really good people, no problem at all as patients, and they adored their little girl. Rightly so. I led them into the room and left them alone, saying I'd be outside if they needed me. It was important they actually saw the body. Nowadays they come in for a little something to help them sleep, and I always give it to them without much probing. They can have whatever they need, as far as I'm concerned.

Conan was fine, physically, except for a lacerated leg. He gave me the story that he swerved to avoid a wallaby. Not likely. There'd been no animal on that road in living memory. Conan was speeding and lost control of the car, and everybody knew it.

He was moaning. 'Why does this always happen to me?'

'Listen mate, quiet down, she's the one who's dead,' I said. He was respon-sible for Nicole's death, and possibly that of his baby brother Jayde, through neglect. That he was weighted down nearly to sinking was obvious, but I had no sympathy left for him.

Conan was never charged or prosecuted, at least in a court of law. The police-man said it was obvious he'd been speeding. 'Might be better for him in the long run if he were charged,' he said with real wisdom. But there were no witnesses.

Conan served me last week at the petrol station, where he still works. He's moved into a tiny apartment and keeps to himself. He gets on with it, in his own way. He does his job and nobody bothers him, but he's still got that look in his eyes that I hate to see, especially on a young person, that look of being awake and sober too often in the early-morning hour of the wolf. It never bodes well.

Whitefella dreaming 1

Tommy MacDonald

New York City. A medical conference boring to the point of stultification. Amaranth Fillet looked as displaced as I felt, so we unimpacted ourselves from a colorectal lecture by the famous AR Pito and disappeared into the bowels of the city. Amaranth immersed herself in the glorious architecture and unearthed obscure Middle Eastern sects. I explored potential markets for artists in the Aboriginal communities in which I was working. One would soon catapult me into my own Dreamtime, my own Alcheringa.

Young Edward the petrol sniffer knocked at my door one night when I was on call for the base clinic, out in the desert near Western Australia. I marked my availability by leaving the white Toyota troop carrier in front of my digs. I was taking an extra turn to spell the Aboriginal health worker and the nursing sister who'd shared the callouts while I was at a conference in New York City. Our locum had pulled out at the last minute.

I peered out into a black night, annoyed at being roused from my bed. All that was visible were two sets of white teeth backing away from the door. The people were quite shy.

'Can you come, doc?' asked Young Edward. 'We've got a sick kid.' He was big and beefy and too slow-moving to play football like a lot of the fellas. One older brother started sniffing petrol and went to the city, and Young Edward's sisters feared the same fate would befall him. They needn't have worried: ultimately he would become Eddie Mayfield, respected elder and artist, but that was down the line in my individual Dreamtime. I'm getting ahead of myself.

'Yes,' I said, and the three of us hopped into the troop carrier and set off to a camp 30 miles to the northwest. They filled me in on the way, leading me to suspect bronchitis in the sick child. We fell silent. As often happens, driving to the outstation took a long time, and the presence of my companions was not intrusive. I'd a lot of time to think. What would I find when I arrived? Would anyone ask me to go to another outstation? The other two outstations were 40 and 60 kilometres past this one, down a dirt road, rough as hell, rocky in places, across a riverbed. I hoped the one solar-powered public phone box each outstation contained would remain unoccupied. It was hard to take a history over the telephone. Someone might ring up at God knows what time of the night, and they always spoke quietly. They might say, 'Jimmy's sick,' and hang up.

The only lights came from my headlights and the stars above. I watched for cattle, which often dotted the side of the road. Usually they'd stand around or run off into the bush, but not always. Once I slowed down and pulled over to the other side of the road, but a small one rushed across the road straight into the passenger's door and broke its neck. Wrecked the door. We ate that.

I punched on the Royal Flying Doctor Service radio to try to pick up anybody talking. We were too far away for any music, but even static was comforting. Into the starry night we drove. The sky was magnificent, a vast sparkling black soup. Perhaps one day, I'd have the time to start painting, an old dream, to try to do justice to the way Mother Nature expressed herself out here. I was hopeless with words, unlike my friend Wayne Cooperville. I suspected he wished to be on the high seas somewhere. Swirling oils, Van Gogh and the smell of turpentine flickered at the tips of my fingers.

When we arrived at the outstation some time later, the dogs all rushed into the headlights, hundreds of them, outnumbering the people. They were a real mixed grill, a Great Dane–type canine, a greyhound, a lot of houndy-looking dogs with pointy noses and ears that stuck up, and little lapdogs and silky terriers. I slowed down to avoid running over not only dogs but also pieces of old car that could puncture the tyres.

One of the men greeted us, grabbed my kit box and walked me across to the patient, through the pungent gidgee wood smoke of the campfire. Gidgee's an acacia with a characteristic aroma, almost offensive, particularly if it's rained. It's a slow-growing, hard desert timber, similar to Tasmanian she-oak, which burns slowly, gives out a lot of heat and leaves only a fine residue of grey ash, not like a eucalyptus.

It was eerie, walking through the smoke and the barking dogs, past the glow of the fire, knowing that people were all round. Two patients I'd seen last week might be among the invisible faces. I'd stitched up a drunken lad who had cracked onto another woman, so his wife hit him in the head with an iron bar or a steel fence dropper. It must have been some party, because somebody stabbed an old chap in the neck. I met them on the road on the way to the outstation and put the lad and the old man into the back of the truck. The elder one was bleeding badly. I resuscitated him, put in a drip, stopped his bleeding and wondered whether he'd survive until the morning: the flying doctor wouldn't come out at night and pick up a drunken person.

Someone threw a few branches on the fire. The light flared, illuminating several people, none of whom I knew. The arc of a torch swung towards me, beckoning me into the darkness. I switched on my own torch. The nights were chilling down, and the child's suspected bronchitis might have developed into pneumonia – a common occurrence in both children and adults in the colder months when the weather plummets to 0°C.

The bloody dogs were nipping at me and sniffing like mad. I stepped on a few unavoidably – mostly – and raised some yelps.

''im not chicky, 'im not chicky,' said one woman, referring to the dogs. 'Cheeky' means bellicose out there. From under her blanket, this woman produced the sick kid I'd been called out to.

Torchlight proved cumbersome, so I turned to my guide. 'Can you switch on the headlights of the troop carrier?' While he was gone, I stuck a thermometer into the girl's mouth and took a history. The dogs sniffed my backside every time I bent over.

"im not chicky, 'im not chicky,' piped a growing chorus of laughing female voices. These women may not have considered their dogs aggressive, but it was bloody terrifying to be bending over from the waist, examining this child's chest and having dogs upon me whose main food was dirty nappies. One bite could cause some damage.

The headlights of the troop carrier acted as searchlights, spotlighting people keeping the wind at bay with old car bonnets and bits of plastic. More plastic appeared when it rained. You watched where you stepped or drove, in case you trod on someone sleeping. This was hard living, in humpies with only a fire and a few dogs to keep warm.

I confirmed the diagnosis of bronchitis. I'd adjusted my expectations out here involving sick children. Choices and decisions awaited. Was it best for the child to stay put and start the treatment immediately? Should I pack people into the vehicle and drive back to the settlement? The family might say not to go back in; they'd no friends or anybody to stay with. I'd have to return the next day to give the girl the next injection or arrange for her to come in. I decided to leave her, knowing that, fortunately, tomorrow was Tuesday, one of our twice-weekly outstation days. We did routine things, like providing medication to hypertensive patients, and some not so routine, like treating kids for pneumonia with intramuscular penicillin for a 5-day course of an appropriate dose, depending on their weight. If my kid had pneumonia, my priority would be regular shots of penicillin. Some of those mothers had competing priorities. If the child improved after, say, day three and the family group was going to another community 100 kilometres away, or if some hunting and gathering was occurring that day, the mother might remove the child partway through the course of penicillin. I would never think, 'Okay, my kid doesn't need its fourth dose of penicillin because we're going down to the supermarket.' Raising people's levels of knowledge to enable informed choices regarding treatment doesn't happen overnight. It's going to take one or two generations. That's one of the reasons why changes in Aboriginal health, well-being, mortality and morbidity are not going to change suddenly.

As the gidgee smoke rose to the stars that night, the little girl's mother thanked me shyly. I was in a pool of light with six or eight adult women lying on the ground and not another child in sight. I looked properly at the sick child's mother. She was immense. A frightening amount of obesity exists, caused by changes in lifestyle and diet and possibly the thrifty gene, which processes carbohydrates and proteins differently than Caucasians and predisposes them to type 2 diabetes.

'Everybody else okay?' I asked.

In a flash, women started popping children out from the blankets like Mandrakes pulling rabbits from hats. White people can't stand the heat and Aborigines can't stand the cold, so by night their teeth chattered and they wrapped blankets round themselves. One of the problems with communities like this was that most people slept in a group outside on the ground to keep warm, so Western medicine was useless. They poked their kids down in-between, and the dogs too. What was the point of treating people for skin infestations if they slept rough with the dogs? I hopped around again as another dog sniffed my backside. It was funny for me even at the time, and people laughed and laughed. Here was this scared white man who jumped and jumped while examining the kids they pulled from the blankets.

I drove back alone, fiddling with the radio, finding company in the static. I dropped over the edge of a shallow escarpment that by day gave a magnificent view of grey and green undulating gidgee and gums stretching across rolling country and a low line of blue hills spiking a massive sky on the horizon.

Next day, I revisited the camp to give the little girl some penicillin and check the other children from the night before. What with one thing and another, the sun was setting by the time I finished at the camp and climbed into the troop carrier. My swag was in the back. I planned to bunk down under the stars and continue to the next outstation in the morning. I did this occasionally, so no one would be alarmed back at base clinic.

I was driving along happily, from a small community of 100 people to a tiny community with 30, on a back track heading west into the setting sun through flat country. I felt safe driving through sand-hill country. Our troop carrier weighed 2 tonnes. A bull bar protected the front. That was fine if you hit something with a low centre of gravity, like a sheep or a kangaroo. Camels were different. Their tall legs, at a metre and a half or two, made their centre of gravity different. Collision would throw one of these desert animals on the vehicle, or over the top if you hit it hard enough. Another risk of isolated areas is having a blowout on a gravel road or sandy track and losing control of the vehicle. Roads are usually firm and dry; when it rains they often become muddy, slippery and boggy. Passing vehicles leave ruts, the rain stops and the sun reappears, the mud bakes as hard as a rock, and you've got problems.

I drove through *tali*[1] country, flat as far as the eye could see, past endless hummocks of dust-coloured spinifex. This grass is similar to pampas but smaller, with tight stalks that are round and razor-sharp on the ends. Spinifex grows outward like a fungal fairy ring, starting in the centre and expanding until a toadstooly ring claims the perimeter. Ghost gums and forests of desert oaks flourished along watercourses, but none were visible at that moment.

Suddenly, a camel loomed out of nowhere. I swerved. The Toyota rolled. I hit a tree and my life changed. The camel catapulted me into my own Alcheringa, which was discrete from Aboriginal ones and whose language and reality were all my own.

In a time of thirsty land when even red dust was too hot to rise, our mob beheld a mud well made by a pale boy driving camels.

---

1 'Sand hill' in several Aboriginal languages.

'I'm back'

Petra Neumann

'Knowing a patient for years does not ensure one's safety, sometimes quite the opposite,' Petra Neumann said. 'The madnesses of everyday life that march through our surgeries are generally not of the mass chainsaw-murdering variety. Usually reputable citizens are going about their daily business when their loved ones or neighbours slip out of gear, usually from drugs, stress or genetics. Something dangerous wriggles through from a parallel reality and turns life as we knew it unliveable, like buying petrol and milk.'

Violence against GPs is nothing new. Tommy MacDonald told me recently about an Aboriginal patient he'd known for years who became a different person when he was sniffing petrol. He'd be dead if he hadn't ducked under a desk and crawled to the door. And that poor Druze doctor in Melbourne, Australia, who was murdered by a patient. And she a woman, like myself. No wonder so many young doctors want to work part-time, preferring quality of life. Are they taking the medical school places of those for whom it is a calling? Where did we take a wrong turn?

Sometimes society lets us down. The dovetailing of two events, a dangerously ill but seemingly normal patient and system failure, can lead to disaster. I barely averted it, and only because I fled the country to the most remote spot I could find. I'll never forget how it all began.

After a detour into psychology, I had settled back into general practice. My days unrolled gently into the far distance.

And then, one afternoon, the telephone rang.

'Doctor!' screamed Mrs Dean. 'I'm afraid he's going to kill me this time! He's got a gun, and he's turning just like his father!'

'I'll be right over.'

'I can't convince him I'm not a communist spy.'

'Try not to disagree with him until I get there.'

'I hate him, doctor!' I heard the resentment that creeps in on the back of too much pain or grief.

'I'm sure you do, and I don't blame you,' I said soothingly. 'I want you to tell me all about it when we've sorted this out.'

'Come round the back.'

'All right.'

'And doctor?'

'Yes?'

'Please hurry!'

The Deans' entire tiny two-roomed weatherboard cottage was miniature. Two stunted fir trees stood sentinel on either side of the veranda at the end of a short walkway. A battered white truck stood near the street end of a gravelled drive, the family vehicle since time immemorial that chauffeured the Deans' twin daughters through their school years. As soon as they could, the girls drove off into oblivion in different vehicles.

I walked down the drive, past rusted oil drums and random piles of bricks. Those fir trees were the only signs of plant life.

Mrs Dean flung open the kitchen door before I knocked. 'He won't listen to anything I say!' No woman on the right side of forty should have that grimness parenthesising her mouth or jerky nervousness to her gait.

Her husband loomed behind her and exclaimed triumphantly, 'I caught her out!' He was a heavyset man of forty-three, too large for his minuscule house. 'She's not normal. The commies sent her over here to meet me. How could I be so stupid?' He hit his brow with a closed fist, hard.

The first thing I did was locate the .22 rifle, which lay on the bench top near the stove.

'I can't win!' Mrs Dean cried, raking hair back behind her left ear with a quick curving motion and patting it down neatly. 'I try not to pressure Ken to earn more and buy me things, and this is my reward. I can't do anything right.'

'She doesn't want a dishwasher,' he said. He pulled the back of his head into alignment with his spinal column. This gave him three chins, like nesting tables.

'Every normal woman wants a dishwasher.'

'Why don't we have a cup of tea, Mr Dean, and we can talk about it.'

'I have to run up to the shops,' Mrs Dean said. 'We're out of milk. I'm sorry, doctor.'

Mr Dean propelled himself at his wife. 'Where the hell do you think you're going, you traitor? You don't fool me.'

'That's enough, Ken,' I said, standing in front of his wife.

'Neither do you.' He raised a threatening arm and looked from one of us to the other. A wicked chuckle of dawning awareness broke the tension. 'You're in this together. I should have known. Bloody doctors. Bloody women.' Paranoid schizophrenics usually have quite complex delusion and bizarre ideas. They are clever enough to know what you are likely to believe and usually don't say anything you can deny or disprove. 'You gave her classified material and now she's going to send it in.'

'Let your wife buy us some milk, Ken. It will give us a chance to talk.'

Mrs Dean was nearly out the door.

'How long will you be gone?'

'I don't know, not long.'

Mr Dean looked at the Mickey Mouse clock above the sink. 'It's 4:23 now. Be back at 4:35. Shouldn't take you more than 12 minutes to walk to the shops and back. That is, of course, if you really *are* going out for milk.'

'Sit down, Ken,' I said as soon as the door slammed.

15

Ken ran to the door and yelled out, 'If you're not back at 4:35, I'm coming after you!' Like so many paranoid schizophrenics, he exploited his wife's desire to please and placate him. He pushed away what he needed desperately and pretended it was her fault. He was only fooling himself.

'Come over here,' I said firmly.

Reluctantly, he lowered himself into a kitchen chair, which was a great relief. I'd not have been able to control the situation if he'd refused. Ken's delusions centred upon the foundry where he worked. They were going to bring in communist agents and machinery that could easily be turned into weapon systems to invade the country. His paranoia included his wife, whom he accused of infidelity, among other things, and reined in tightly.

'This is a fine mess, Ken. We've got a real problem.' I put myself on his side, rather than saying, 'You've got a problem.'

'Why are you so interested?'

'Because you are *both* my patients. Look at what your behaviour has achieved. You've driven your wife to the edge of despair.'

'I knew you were in this with that bitch!'

'What do you mean?' I put my best effort into sounding puzzled.

'She always throws your name at me.'

I changed tacks. 'I think you're carrying a heavy burden, Ken. Can you tell me what problems you're experiencing?'

'Nobody is supposed to know, but I found out,' he whispered, visibly relaxing. He leaned forward conspiratorially and added, 'Certain people here are in league with the communists. It's my duty to do something.' Suddenly, he looked suspicious. 'What's this to do with you?'

'I want to be fair and I want to hear all your complaints. I don't want your views to go unheard.' That usually is reasonably disarming to people. They do want to air their side.

In my experience, many schizophrenics become extremely confrontational because they don't feel anybody hears them out. If you can air all their ideas, you may find a complicated system of delusions behind the obvious one, which can be that 'My wife doesn't love me', or 'She's wasting money' or 'She's hoarding money for herself.' Many many times I've been enmeshed in terrible marital disputes, heard appalling stories from the wife. The husband's in a right fighting mood. If I were to say, 'Your wife tells me this and that', he'd tell me to fuck off and be highly aggressive. Most people respond if I say, 'I can't *believe* that's the complete story.'

'Is it some problem between you and your wife?'

'Fuck off.'

'I *need* to have your side as well, Ken.' I was very, very careful not to raise the level of confrontation, of anger.

'She used to be totally controlled by someone on that radio programme on the ABC.'

'Why do you think a broadcasting company is controlling her?'

'She listens to it all the time. They must be sending her messages. And she's in league with the communists.'

'What evidence do you have for this?'

'I found a commie newspaper in the house.'

Mr Dean seized upon a small strand of evidence upon which to build his plot. To me, it was enough, along with the communist and radio programmes, to be able to say, *This person's got psychotic ideas.* He'd turn dangerous unless I threaded successfully through a verbal minefield. Ken seemed to have forgotten the .22 on the bench top.

'. . . and through the foundry,' Ken was saying.

'That's where you work, isn't it?'

This was when people in the West feared that communists were behind all bad things. The Berlin Wall had just come down and the Cold War ended. Mr Dean's factory had recently bought a lot of machinery from Eastern Europe, probably a source of cheaper goods than that available from a Western ally. He felt that the origin of these materials meant the entire management of the company was communist. His wife – as was usual in these cases, when he got into conflict with her over something quite simple, and it could be anything – was added to this complex paranoid system of ideas. Paranoia is a feature of only some schizophrenia. Many many *many* of my schizophrenic patients have not annexed such complex paranoid ideas, and perhaps experience only a minimal degree of disturbance, including disintegration in their social skills and performance. They might stop looking after themselves and neglect their room and their work, or become remote and hear voices that order them to do things.

'Yeah, that's my workplace. Don't you understand?' he asked with incredible urgency. 'I've *seen* them talking. That's a cover. They're planning how to bring in agents. I've observed them bringing in that *machinery,* they call it, *for the foundry,*' he mimicked with bitter scorn. 'They can't fool me! They can turn that stuff into weapons systems. I have to do something before they overrun the country!'

Certifying Mr Dean was inevitable. He was clearly a risk to himself and the community, not to mention his wife.

'Mr Dean, do you have any proof?'

'Proof!' he gloated. 'I'll show you! Come with me.'

I noticed a telephone nearby. 'I'd rather wait here, if that's okay with you.'

'Please yourself,' he shrugged.

The moment Mr Dean was out the door I ran to the telephone. By the time he returned, the police were on the way.

It was 4:34. He glowered at the Mickey Mouse clock. 'She's only got 1 minute!'

At 4:36, he shouted, 'That bitch! I knew I shouldn't have let her out of my sight! I'll kill her!'

I prayed the police would come quickly. A few minutes later, a fist pounded at the door.

Ken looked over, scowling.

'Police! Open up!'

'Come in now!' I cried.

Ken was at the bench top in a flash, grabbing the .22. Fortunately, two fit law enforcement officers pinned him down before he inflicted any damage.

'You betrayed me, you rotten bitch!' he screamed at me as he struggled.

'Ken, you really ought to be in hospital for a rest.'

'*She* bribed you, didn't she?'

'Calm down, mate,' said one policeman.

'These men will take you, so you don't have to drive yourself.'

As I was climbing into my car, Mrs Dean peeked out from a hiding place on the side of the garage, milk in hand. 'I'll ring the hospital psychiatrist from the surgery and do the necessary,' I assured Mrs Dean. 'Will you be all right?'

She nodded.

'Come to the surgery in the morning.'

She was my first patient the next day. We were both shaken by the events of the day before and yearned for the stage of leisurely discussion, threat past.

'At first, I liked it when Ken always wanted to know where I was and when I was coming home,' Mrs Dean said. Her movements were jerky. 'So many men don't care what you do. But things got out of hand. He started ringing round my friends every 10 minutes and turning up at their houses. He frightened them.'

'He's safely locked away and can do no harm.'

'I hope so, doctor.'

'Did anything specific happen at work?'

'Not that I know of. That's another thing I noticed: he insisted on knowing exactly where I was all the time, but if I asked him about his day, he got suspicious and asked me why I wanted to know. Whenever I ask him to talk to you, it blows up in my face.'

I recalled Ken's accusations and looked at her for a long moment. 'He's very sick, Mrs Dean.'

I think many GPs experience heartsink when they see a schizophrenic patient. Initially, schizophrenics' abnormalities are not immediately clear. You may wait a long time for a clue to the pathology. One day, they step over a border and you think, 'This is clearly psychotic behaviour. They have bizarre ideas and disordered mentation.' It's obvious if a patient presents as Jesus Christ back on earth or Muhammad recreated. I've always found female schizophrenics less violent than male ones, like one young girl. She was actually quite bizarre. She constructed the most amazing meanings around what I perceived as insignificant events, like a light bulb shattering. Once she told me that the way the pieces fell on the floor indicated a major sexual connotation. Because the light bulb shattered in this explicit sexual way, she'd have to do this and that. She wrote me a letter. 'Now that this has come to be, what should I do? I know you probably won't understand, but I have to do something about it and I'll go outside for some vegetables.' How different she was from an axe-wielding young man whose schizophrenia was ignorantly exacerbated when his family included him in its marijuana enterprises. And how different they both were from Mr Kenneth Dean, also a letter writer.

Ken Dean's schizophrenia was nothing new, but its complexity was expanding, for instance in the web of people enmeshed in his paranoid ideas. He'd not even been diagnosed. His wife had catalogued his descent since I started at the practice, but as he'd been physically robust we'd not been able to persuade him to come to the surgery.

'I can't give him any more, doctor.' She whimpered, exhausted. 'He's used up my love. I tried and I tried and I tried to make him happy.'

'If you have feelings left for him, don't let him come out of hospital to an empty home. That might send him over the edge. Give me some time to get him into the system.'

She looked irresolute. 'All right, doctor,' she said wearily, hooking her hair behind her left ear and patting it down.

Later that morning, I was on my way home to lunch when the phone rang. 'He's out,' Mrs Dean whispered.

'Already!' I cried.

A wail of pain was followed by an unpleasant snicker. 'Yeah, I sweet-talked them shrinks.' Mr Dean must have grabbed the telephone from his wife. '"Nothing's wrong with Mr Dean," I told 'em. "He's only sick of his wife. She's been giving him a hard time and he was only returning it." They all understood *that*. I'm coming for you, doc.'

With that, the phone slammed down.

They let him out at half past eleven, and at 12:00 noon he'd been home and got a gun and was looking for me. I rang the consulting psychiatrist immediately. 'Mr Dean is an extremely dangerous man. I have no doubt he'd have killed me if he'd seen me,' I said, and explained what happened.

'Oh yeah, he was probably worse than we realised,' he said offhandedly.

'It was a *great* mistake, very very wrong and totally negligent, to have let him out so quickly.'

He expressed neither embarrassment nor concern that they'd released him.

'I can understand that you found no reason to keep him in, but I think it was irresponsible that you didn't ring up and tell me. In that event, I'd have seen him in hospital and said, "Look, I'd like you to go home," as if I were taking part in the decision and not let him be sent out with the idea that I was the problem.'

The system let me down. A major row ensued between the psychiatrist and myself. 'I think the whole department behaved irresponsibly,' I said. 'I am no longer prepared to be part of a system that is run so unsatisfactorily. You can remove me from the list of doctors you call upon to go out and certify patients.'

We got Ken readmitted to the psychiatric hospital, where he stayed for a long time.

Other patients and problems presented themselves and I forgot the Deans, until the phone rang one day. 'It's Mrs Dean, doctor. I want you to know that I'm really leaving. Thank you very much for all you've done.' She took the family car, sold all the possessions in the house and disappeared interstate.

This story has a postscript. As Dr Nicky Doulton-Brown says, there's something to be said for neighbourhoods. Paddy the mechanic prevented a tragedy because he knew two people: myself and the man after me with a gun. I was returning to work one day from lunch. I called in to fill up the car and purchase some milk for work. The petrol station was two blocks past the surgery on the road out of town.

'A guy's been looking for you. He's got a gun in his car and is threatening to shoot you,' Paddy said.

'Do you know who it is?'

'Yeah doc, that guy from the foundry. You just missed him. He was acting strangely. He waved a gun and kept asking, "Have you seen Dr Neumann?" I said you were away on holidays.'

'Thanks, Paddy, you saved my life.'

I immediately returned home. On the way, I saw 'I'm back' scrawled nearly illegibly in red paint across the front of our surgery. I prayed that Mrs Dean had well and truly disappeared.

I phoned the police as soon as I walked through my door. They picked him up and found a loaded shotgun in his car. The psychiatric hospital readmitted him. Once again, the psychiatrist expressed no remorse, only, 'He was probably worse than we thought.'

Mr Dean is so paranoid that even now, after all these years, he finds me wherever I'm practicing and writes threatening letters. He even photographs the surgery, to show that he knows where I am. 'You're one of their agents and I can get you anytime I want,' he says. He probably goes on medication, becomes reasonably well behaved, and stops. That's the usual pattern.

Ken traced his wife interstate in the end. Whenever a domestic tragedy hits the news, I wonder if he's finally killed the wife who tried to love him.

Samurai swords and ▬ tongue-lashings

Nicky Doulton-Brown

Trail of ex-wives. Waiting in a sport utility vehicle in the parking lot of a massive shopping mall for my pregnant daughter by my fourth spouse. We all assumed that was it. No one was more surprised than I when she ended it, after years of an armed truce born of intertwined vested interests. I remember my home visits to the area when this mall was a real neighbourhood, with cared-for houses and tended people. Over by that department store was Mrs O'Reilly's house. I was able to out-manipulate her once and still regret it.

That autumn Monday morning, something made me stop at Mrs Dymphna O'Reilly's on my way to Thalia Skurley next door. Perhaps it was the familiar fluttering of the bedroom's lace curtains that trumpeted a lurking inquisitive resident. In vain, I fought the temptation to check on the old duck. It was a quarter to eight and it certainly wasn't Tuesday. She insisted on 'Eight o'clock of a Tuesday morning, doctor, and only then.'

Mrs O'Reilly manipulated everybody, all her healthcare contingent as well as her family. Tuesday morning was when the doctor came, Tuesday afternoon the nurse rolled up and Wednesday it was somebody else. It was all quite elaborately plotted. She got very cross if you said to her, 'I can't come on Tuesday, but I'll be coming on Wednesday.' Standards had to be maintained. We were only allowed to examine the old lady in her bed at 8:00 in the morning because she was blowed if she was going to undress during the rest of the day. She'd been widowed around the time of the First World War. I doubted she'd disrobed for any man since, and possibly not ever. She never remarried.

The extent of my blunder soon became clear. I felt ashamed of the zing humming along my nerve endings as I strutted up the path on my way to foil an adversary. Hah.

'Mrs O'Reilly?' I sang out in my best morning voice. I let myself into the house.

I heard aggrieved scrambling and sighing in the bedroom. And something else. My ears must be playing up. Patients never told one to go away. I opened the bedroom door, which I'll regret to my dying day.

'You're early, doctor, and it's Monday.' Mrs O'Reilly was wigless and obviously mortally offended that I'd glimpsed her wispy strands. She was bending over a chest of drawers whose open middle disgorged a jumble of hair, all of it white and some of it with curls of blue, pink and lavender.

'I was just . . .' I began, feebly. I still recall the horror, resentment and vulnerability in her red-rimmed eyes. I'd transgressed. We both knew it.

She climbed into bed. That this tidy woman left her wig drawer hanging open underscored her confusion. I'd deprived her of what little control and dignity remained. To such depths had I sunk. She chattered on and on, ending with complaints about the neighbours. I saw it so often. What a great word is *complain*, with so many animal synonyms: beef, bitch, carp, grouse.

I finally broke in to ask, 'How have you been, Mrs O'Reilly?'

'Attended one of those Tupperware parties yesterday, doctor, up at the top end,' she said. The glow of disgust permanently creased the right side of her face. 'One of the two ex-military wives at the top end invited most of the neighbours. Even that poor mousy thing down the bottom end came.' I knew the family. It required courage for that poor soul, so beaten down and up by life, to venture the gauntlet of the street.

A great gulf lay between the ladies in the use to which they put those plastic bowls and tight-fitting lids. Those from the law-and-order end of the street stored cakes in them, which were made from recipes precisely torn from women's magazines and pasted into personal notebooks. My patient gestured across the street with her head and said, '*She* stores marijuana in her Tupperware, and you know how fresh it keeps everything. Loathsome.'

In this case, the widow's derisions received scientific validation. It is well known that people from neighbouring communities can find each other's habits revolting. Work in the field shows that women are more easily disgusted than men, an emotion that traditionally wards off contamination.[2] If disgust motivates avoidance of contact in order to reduce exposure to pathogens and toxins,[3] then old Mrs Dymphna O'Reilly was impaled on the horns of a dilemma, wedged between the rock-and-rolling Skurleys and a pious, attentive church lady whose only sin was compulsive lying. Both the rockers and the sanctified were the souls of kindness to Mrs O'Reilly, and she couldn't stand them. She suffered the great misfortune not to approve of any of her neighbours. It had nothing to do with age and everything to do with sensibility. Shotgun-toting ferals resided across the road – I understood her disapproving of *them* – rendering them too far away to matter. So far had her world constricted. She didn't know, as I did from the nurse who visited twice a week, that they were not complying with their tuberculosis medication regime and consequently were in no state to shoot at any of their neighbours' garden gnomes.

'Something's wrong with that Skurley lad, always going off to that shed behind the house. Must be full of drugs.'

'He's a rock star, Mrs O'Reilly, and he built that soundproofed shed for his practice sessions.'

'He's disgusting.'

2 Fessler *et al.* 2004.
3 Ibid. p. 6.

'What exactly do you find offensive?'

'Well, his hair for one thing. And those swords he keeps bringing in. Mark my words, one day he'll use them on his poor wife. So clean, she is.'

I looked at my watch. 'Other patients are waiting, Mrs O'Reilly, so we'd better start. How have you been this week?'

The consultation was unremarkable. I examined Mrs O'Reilly through a ruffled dressing gown, surrounded by photographs of a dashing young man in his army uniform. Normally, I find photographs a great way of uncovering extra bits of family and medical history. That gallant soldier stared out of his frame and across half a century to reproach me.

I'd not the same spring in my step when I latched the gate behind me on the way out. No marks for surprising a vulnerable old woman whom I'd not allowed to don her physical or psychological armour. I'd won this round – perhaps – but at what cost? I was ashamed of myself.

Such was my state of mind as I unlatched the street gate next door. The resident rock star was a man with obsessions, ones that would have remained undetected had I seen him only in the surgery. He made sculptures out of old tyres, peeling them this way and that to unleash the black-and-white swans within. Rusted-out car hulks fortified the front yard, arranged like a battery of tanks protecting the swans. Inside this phalanx of concrete monstrosities a mini-community thrived: an Aborigine with a spear, a porpoise, a sheep, two chickens and three elves. All bore signs of gunfire. The family on the other side of the street especially liked leaning out the front window and taking potshots with a .22 at the concrete gnomes.

That day, I stopped to pay respects to the fallen piccaninnies and dolphins riddled with bullet holes. The man of the house cracked the front door open and beckoned me inside a decaying weatherboard house.

'Thanks for coming,' he said, flicking the kiss curl of his long, dyed black hair out of his eyes. Like his neighbour Mrs O'Reilly's, the right side of Shep's mouth contorted into a permanent sneer, but his had nothing to do with disgust. Elvis Presley incarnate.

'You're welcome, Shep.'

'It's Thalia, doc,' he said in a curiously high-pitched voice, evoking an image of his beautiful, well-dressed wife. He hunched forward and rabbited ahead with disturbed, anxious steps. As I knew from previous home visits, he was terrified of cancer. Each symptom must be the Big C.

I followed Shep over a knot of fallen umbrellas and round a bicycle, down a passageway dim in the morning light. Movie posters, album jackets and promotional photographs smothered the walls. All displayed images of Elvis, either as embattled prisoner in *Jailhouse Rock*, lei-laden king of rock in *Blue Hawaii* or smilingly sanitised on his Christmas album, the one with the bright-red background. I brushed against three more images. Singer as bloated Las Vegas lounge lizard, early Elvis mourning the dog Old Shep before he dyed his hair black and contented husband eating fried banana-and-peanut-butter sandwiches at Graceland.

'Look at this.' Shep the rocker lifted his arm. His sleeve fell back. Tattoos shrouded every square centimetre of skin. 'Great innit, doc? That's me favourite.'

He pointed to Elvis in black leather on a motorcycle looking self-consciously surly.

A middle-aged woman and a massive young man obviously cut from the same genetic cloth approached from the kitchen-cum-lounge into which the passage widened at the back.

'You remember my wife's mother and brother, doc?' He introduced them and faded away.

'Hello, Mrs Stephanides,' I said to a woman barely 4 feet tall, with bad teeth and grey threads through her black hair.

'This way, doctor. Stay here,' she ordered her son. He nodded with those large Hellenic eyes that look languid or leering.

We ducked into a room on the left near the front of the house, past the Elvis posters. Thalia Skurley sometimes attended the surgery for menorrhagia. I wondered if she was having trouble with her periods again. Shep had adroitly married an elegant Greek girl with beautifully coiffed hair and fabulous clothes. She always shimmied in looking a million dollars.

My expectations collided with reality on that home visit. I kicked a path through knickers, pantyhose and other female undergarments, which lost all allure when cast upon the floor. I cleared the way to the bed with my feet. How could such a neat and tidy lady have such a shambolic bedroom?

'What seems to be the problem, Thalia?' I said and glanced meaningfully at the mother, which she was supposed to interpret as a signal to leave. In the best of all worlds. Instead, she overrode her daughter's tentative squeaks and said, 'It's her period again, doctor.'

'I'd prefer to examine Thalia alone, Mrs Stephanides.'

The elder woman grimaced and left the room.

Who invented waterbeds? They are guaranteed to raise our chances of being sued for malpractice.

'What's wrong?' I repeated, leaning forward.

She lay just beyond grasping range. Blades of hair grazed her biceps.

Her eyes twisted in pain as she caressed her abdomen lightly with her fingertips. Her eyes were as big as her brother's, but her nose and lips were small, imparting a vulnerable beauty.

'Where exactly is the pain?'

She poked her lower right abdomen.

Ever graceful, I applied knee to waterbed as I tried to palpate her.

Thalia bounced up and down like a basketball. I nearly lost my balance. She smiled faintly.

'Is the pain dull?'

She shook her head.

'Sharp?'

'Sometimes.'

'Does it hurt when you cough?'

'No.'

'Do you feel it anyplace else, like your back or leg?'

Another shake of the head.

I was fairly certain about Thalia's diagnosis: a bad case of menstrual cramps. I wanted to confirm it. The action of moving to palpate Thalia's abdomen rolled her towards the centre of the bed. Up shot my grounding leg, onto the waterbed.

'Bowel action today?'

'No.'

'Yesterday?'

'Think so.'

'How's your appetite?'

'Okay.'

Thalia kept moving farther and farther away from me as I palpated her.

'Have you been sexually active – oh!'

I fell on top of her, squarely and completely, and thought, 'Oh my God! Her brother's going to come in. He's Greek and he'll kill me!' Her husband the Elvis clone didn't bother me. The harder I endeavoured to regain a dignified medical position, the more we rolled around.

'Thalia!' I cried.

'Oh, doctor!'

My life flashed before my eyes. I was certain that Mama would burst in, dressed all in black, waving a camera. I would be paying for the rest of my life. Finally, I climbed off the waterbed on all fours, like a terrier treading water. I fell on the beige pile carpet and noticed several mouldy McDonald's chips under the bed, bent and spent.

'Thalia,' I said with gravity. 'You have a severe case of menstrual cramps.'

She looked at me from the centre of that bloody waterbed and giggled.

After the appropriate ministrations, I retraced my steps through the debris on the floor. I glanced through various open doors on my way down the hallway. The rest of the house was equally shambolic. Discord reigned here, except for the Elvis posters geometrically aligned. I strode towards the beckoning smells of sweet syrup and bitter coffee, passed a collage of the King's army days and entered the kitchen/living area at the back of the house. Mother, brother and husband, all lounging in various states of relaxation, snapped to as I entered. I sketched Thalia's prognosis and treatment, omitting details of what was a private consultation, not a family affair.

'I must go,' I said finally. I'd one last call before returning to work and a full load of patients.

'No no, you'll have some something before you go,' Mrs Stephanides ordered, rising. 'Won't be long.'

'C'mon, I want to show you something while we wait.' Shep led me from the kitchen to the living area, hidden by a rice-paper screen. 'I toured in Japan once and caught a bug, but not one you can cure.' His chins bobbed as he chuckled.

'Look!' His hands arced in an opening fan as he gestured at the walls. Samurai swords adorned all spare wall space. 'These here are decorative, me wall hangers. They were straight, not curved, before the year 987. Look at this – real steel, and grain marks you can see. And this one: you can tell it's old because of all the rust on the tang, the bit of the blade inside the *tsuka*, the handle. Cost me, these did.'

I examined a lot of people with arsenals of guns, but never such a collection of knives.

'That bug left me with a permanent love of Japanese sword arts. My favourite's called kendo. We do it with a partner so it's full contact, but less martial than *iaido*, which is done alone. Here,' he added, patting proprietarily a large locked cabinet. 'These are my functional swords for cutting. Light, medium and heavy. They're not made of stainless steel like the decorative ones, but high-carbon steel, with full tangs so the blade can't come loose, and no rattling fixtures. And me practice ones. These two are wooden – carved from an oar and from white oak – and this one, called *shinai*. Can you guess what it's made from?'

'Haven't a clue,' I said.

'Bamboo! Four slats, bound with string and leather. It's safer than the wooden ones because it's light and flexible. Notice the oval grip. It's more traditional than the round one. We use *shinai* a lot in kendo, and I use it onstage in my act. My fans love it. We build up to that cracking sound when striking an opponent. Elvis would have approved. We mike up the bass player so I don't have to hit him hard, and he hams it up.'

'Amazing,' I said truthfully. This man kept revealing obsession after obsession. The Big C. Tyre swans. Elvis Presley and now samurai swords. I judged that he wouldn't use the last in anger. Later I was proven wrong, and not for the first time.

'Here, boys!' cried Mama Stephanides. To her, any male of any age was a boy.

We dutifully descended upon the well-scrubbed wooden kitchen table, now laden with huge chunks of home-made baklava and tiny cups of coffee sludge.

I wish I'd accepted the other offerings of those times with better grace. Such generosity decreased as times changed. What this fear-ridden man did to that table years later sent me to plumb the depths of a rock star's anger.

Fried brains and the Polish corpse

Amaranth Fillet

'Let's ride the wave of this coffee buzz and talk about men,' she said, as the sun sank over the seaside bistro. 'Hubby Wayne was singing "Harbor Lights" the night we met, complete with foghorn. It was pure 1950s longing. I loved it. Did you know the Platters' manager was a paleface called Buck Ram?' Layers of sunshine shot through sheets of clouds, like a celestial poppy-seed and apricot torte. 'Look at that sky. Can't you just see a baby unicorn poking through its eggshell? Something hatched in my heart when Wayne crooned "tender nights beside the silvery sea."' She swirled the sludge in her thimble-sized brass cup. 'This is the only drug I allow myself these days. It works for now, not like when I started out.'

The driver wheezed like an old horse. Animal man: bear paws, beefy face, pig eyes. 'A lass your age should be planning for bairns, not cairns,' he snuffled. Woman as stock. Moo. 'Not a chance,' I said airily. I was finished with men, especially after what happened with my pusher. I was going straight, and that was that. Uncle Zoltan spouted Dr Dalrymple at me – bring it on, Theodore – so it was time to assume personal responsibility for my choices. I couldn't let Uncle Z down again. He'd have understood and simply lectured me as he buffed his buttery loafers. Which would've made it worse.

I contemplated leaving medicine for a cloistered existence, but realised I was built for speed, like Long Tall Sally. I was determined to stop meaning *that* kind of speed. It was all intertwined with men. So long, Commonwealth male. Been round the block a few times with the standard-issue sedan. Took me nowhere. The sports model took me too far in the wrong direction. Traded it in for space on a passenger jet and three bus, boat and ferry rides. Beef up the career with variety. Hello, mother country. Moo, long before bovine spongiform encephalopathy, commonly known as mad cow disease. Merry old England and all her islands, some of them wondrously remote.

During my pre-Wayne wanderings, I did a locum for a friend on an island off an island off an island. Working for her senior partner was supposed to straighten my head. Surely *there* I'd have no temptations. According to Petra

Neumann, so had supposed the island's previous doctor, the one they carted off for alcoholism. And the mad one before that, who got himself and his horse permanently stuck in Doctors Bog, where they were turning to peat. My indiscretions seemed minor, and I'd the excuse of youth.

Because of Petra's newborn babe, I lodged with the Nesbitts for my 3-month locum: Jimmy, Fiona and their two children, an X and a Y. Chromosomes, that is. Girl and boy. Talk about landing in other people's marital minefields! Jimmy Nesbitt and his wife coexisted in orgasmic acrimony. Jimmy picked me up from the airstrip, a compact model striding towards me propelled by eyebrows like rusty bullets. Mother Nature compensated Jimmy's lack of height with a breathtakingly handsome face, which he buried under a gravity-defying ZZ Top–type coppery beard. 'Some of us can play at saving the world,' he scowled. Arsenic model. He clawed his iron fingers through strawberry hair that began profusely in the middle of his head and ended spent and limp on his shoulders. 'You can. You're a women's libber.' (Wild guess.) 'The wife can. All Fiona has to do is open her bloody mouth and warble. Me, I have Responsibilities, a family to support. Living here is bloody hard work. I make sacrifices so we can stay. I can't paint, not half as much as I want. I have to run the bloody ferry service and work as a handyman. Me!'

Such was my chest-beating introduction to those idyllic isles, a foretaste of stranger fruit dangling from the non-poplar trees, sparse as they were. Sing it Billie!

'C'mon, you're staying with us. I'll take you to meet the wife. We don't live far.'

The wife. Fiona's looks ranged from engaging to equine, depending upon the way she held her receding chin. She 'did' at the Big House and drove the manager's wife demented by dusting in great sweeping arcs without moving furniture or curios, earnestly folk-singing all the while. No one else would do the work, and Fiona Nesbitt knew it. Tyranny plus.

Four weeks in, I did a callout of which I have not the slightest recollection. No, no, don't worry, drugs weren't involved, not that anything beckoned from that chronically understocked and out-of-date supply cabinet. I'd checked it out on my first day.

The day began at 4:00 in the morning with Fiona as hostess trilling in that lilt for which the islanders were famous, 'A bit of breakfast afore ye go, doctor?'

I knew what *that* meant: boiled penguin eggs, battered testicles and brain fritters. I never quite *got* boiled penguin eggs. The white is transparent and surrounds a red-orange ball, which stares at you after you cut the top off. The whole thing is huge and smells overpoweringly fishy. Battered sheep's testicles were a real speciality. Even sweeping aside my aversion to the actual food – which I was unable to do – the violent adjective stopped me short. Imagine chinless Fiona warbling as she raised and lowered a hammer. Even the vision of an efficient farm wife dunking the pendants in a decoction of flour, water and eggs and dropping them to sizzle in a frying pan overwhelmed me, considering what the poor animal contributed to the occasion. At 4:00 in the morning, it was definitely out. And fried brains, well, I'll *never* get that.

I downed a cup of strong tea by the light of a peat fire. I can't stomach breakfast chit-chat and was thankful now for two things: that the talented Fiona's pragmatism prevented her from being offended ('If she was 'ungry, she would heat'), and that her children were sulkily taciturn. Jimmy was elsewhere.

'You'll be round the settlements if you're needed?' Fiona asked, flipping a fritter in the iron skillet.

I nodded. 'I'll be spending a few days taking human blood for a hydatid survey, based at McDonald's croft.'

Later, I sat at another kitchen table writing on a label. A half-full chipped teacup waited near a picked-at plate of battered sheep's testicles. Charles admonished me that we never knew what the day would bring, and I'd better have something in my stomach to keep my diagnostic abilities oiled. I'd have to live with the consequences the rest of my life. His words gave breakfast a certain allure. I sawed in half and swallowed two cojones, eyes closed.

Senior partner Charles was warming his hands at the fire and declaiming in the tone of someone accustomed to commanding attention. I tuned him out, as advised by my friend Petra. We weren't far from the sea. No place was. The waves seemed to crash in the garden, if you could so call one stunted rosebush.

Suddenly, frantic pounding at the front door accompanied by cries of 'Doctor! Doctor!' rent the tranquillity.

'Better get ready,' Charles ordered, rubbing his hands against his thighs. He strode out of the room.

I heard urgent mutterings. '. . . newly arrived Polish shipping vessel . . . We put the body in the freezer, doc . . . You there! Boatmen! We need two of you!'

Charles shot back into the room. 'Your first callout to a foreign vessel! Come on!'

Heavy seas beckoned, and before 6:00. 'Why? Why is a corpse so urgent?'

'I'll come with you the first time. Hurry!'

One islander hoisted me aboard the small boat taking us to the ship. My stomach rebelled at first whiff as the wind blew the aroma of the brain fritters Charles devoured for breakfast into my face. I envied his ability to eat anything placed before him, no matter what the hour or the delicacy. Thank God I avoided the chains of alcoholism that hobbled so many of my colleagues.

Dawn stained the sky as we set out. Huge great cliffs cut sheets of shadows deep into the big seas. We bobbed along on top, cutting no neat incision in the water. I beheld the only patch of trees, a couple of stunted acres, as we motored away. The rest was rock, rock, rock. The prevailing wind sheared the treetops flat, bequeathing a barren beauty.

Only some of the small surrounding islands we passed were inhabited. Many were single-family islands. Huge great sea cliffs and big rolling seas dominated the Western Isles. Low shorelines rimmed the eastern islands, bisected by large mountains of exposed schist that glinted in the sunshine and glistened when wet.

One of those moments of Spontaneous Stocktake descended when I was literally rocking and rolling. I said before that I chose to spell a friend by doing a locum here, but the truth is that both my medical and familial establishments determined that 3 months – and maybe longer – of practicing in a remote location with a low temptation factor would be best for their errant young 'un. I'd be mortified if I had any shame. Not me. Those finer feelings disappeared with my first pusher. I dared to dream they were only dormant. Encountering endgame – sozzled senior partner – helped enormously. No way would I allow my mind to melt like the churned cream of Uncle Zoltan's shoes.

I was at a crossroads, and I knew it.

Kicks came in unexpected ways. My family hoped further training in a conventional career might provide a few. They weren't far off. I did the most amazing things in those islands. The week before, a forces helicopter flew me miles offshore in hideous weather to administer aid to a sailor in the bottom of a trawler. We almost ran out of fuel. *Just* made it back to shore. Lesson Number One: there's more than one way to get high. I loved it. Underlying it all, beneath the miasma of self-absorption, was my desire to be of benefit to others. That precious jewel was encrusted and needed an energetic burnish.

An approaching storm blowing brittle and mean jerked me back into the present. Pellets of rain pummelled my cheeks. Our skiff nipped at a rolling mountain of water, a terrier riding a tsunami. I didn't look up. The undulating iron-grey water beckoned to the battered testicles I'd downed to vacate my body. 'Wonder what happened to this chap,' I said, to distract myself from the breakfast that was on the move.

'Probably hit by heavy machinery, or possibly a heart attack, like poor old JB,' Charles replied, showing not the slightest ill effects from all those brain fritters. 'I certified JB last time his fleet was here. Died from shock, I wrote. He'd been in a rowing boat underneath a massive whaler, chipping at paint.'

'*That* heart attack would not have been caused by being overweight or leading a sedentary lifestyle,' I said.

'It was weight all right,' Charles retorted. 'Someone dropped the anchor mistakenly. It landed on him.'

I grabbed the flank of the boat as we rolled. Breakfast shifted to the other side of my gut.

'I'll miss him,' Charles said. 'We had some times.'

I knew alcoholic sentimentality when I swayed towards it. Not that the locals drank much alcohol: the blokes were too busy and peer pressure too strong. If they didn't pull their own weight, they and their families would starve. Nobody helped a waster. This was no place for malingerers. The islanders occasionally drank after work, but most alcohol-related trouble involved imported labourers.

Soon the horizon dipped to reveal the Polish fleet. 'These chaps have not seen a woman in months, Dr Fillet,' Charles said.

'Not a problem, if I look half as bad as I feel,' I mumbled.

Soon we bobbed furiously alongside the hull of a ship. A ladder appeared, lowered by strong hands, and a ruddy face peeked over the rim. The face was saying something, which the wind carried away.

They all looked at me. 'Ladies first, doctor,' said my colleague. 'You have to crawl up this ladder.' I looked at the flimsy bit of rope and meagre metal crossbars. What if my feet slipped in the salt spray? Would my arms be strong enough to haul me upwards?

I made it, somehow, not at my most graceful. Ruddy Face pulled me up and over onto the deck. His curious and desperate mates joined him. While Charles negotiated those slippery metal bars, the Polish seamen and I evaluated one another with maximum politeness, as much as their deprived state allowed. I was relieved to feel Charles' bulk behind me, cutting the wind.

Glasses of vodka appeared.

'I can't drink this,' I muttered fiercely to Charles.

'You have to,' he replied. 'They will be totally offended if you do not drink their vodka.'

'I . . . Cannot . . . Drink . . . This,' I repeated. 'It's 6:00 in the morning, and I don't drink vodka anyway.'

'You have to, otherwise your credibility is gone.' Charles chugged down Drink Number One. 'You'll be coming out to these ships, and coming on your own, so you have to drink the vodka.'

Apparently, I got pulled off the boat around 9:00. I can't recall a thing. I woke up in the sisters' bedroom in the hospital at 2:00 in the afternoon with the most almighty hangover. I felt absolutely wretched, having consumed three massive doses of potato-based distilled spirit.

Charles filled in the details later.

'Sounds like we'd better do a post-mortem,' I said.

'We'll see,' Charles replied.

As often happens, they stored the body in the freezer with the fish, the meat, the veggies and the ice cream, right down in the bottom of the ship's hold, so that was where our procession headed.

Normally, doing a post-mortem presupposed no freezing and immediate action – but in the situation described, folk had no option.

Just as well. You can't do a post-mortem only a few hours after the body comes out of a freezer, because it takes ages to thaw. You've got to be able to saw through the tissue if you open up the body parts – head, chest, stomach, etc. The ideal time to do it was before freezing, which obviously can't be done if the body is on a 'mother ship' three or more days' sailing from the nearest port. Freezing preserves the body as it was when frozen – so you can distinguish, for instance, a blow to the head or a stab wound to the chest wall – but some of the organs putrefy rapidly after thawing, like the gut, so definitive statements on those types of organs are very difficult. Often death on ships results from trauma or a heart attack or occasionally stroke.

Charles told me that the seamen were not able to find a body bag, so they wrapped it up in old sails – a common solution – and carefully lowered it over the side of the ship. Our two boatmen received it without a mishap in the rolling seas – a feat of no mean skill. Hitting the water would have sunk it. They piled my warm, limp body atop the stiff, frozen corpse for the return journey. Mercifully, I remembered nothing.

A swinging beam hit the poor bloke on the head, a common cause of death in this hazardous life. I can hazily recall that I agreed most solemnly with my senior partner. No need for a post-mortem.

After that, I always wore Wellingtons on my outings to the ships. I issued many medical clearances and certifications, and always poured the vodka or drink of choice down the side of my rubber boots, otherwise no way could I have remained upright, not offend the sailors and keep it together.

One morning as I was winding down that island gig, the telephone rang at the surgery.

'Perhaps, pet, this was a bad idea after all,' said the one man who never let me down.

'Uncle Zoltan!'

'The image of you climbing swaying rope ladders into foreign vessels and drinking yourself silly is not one I cherish.'

'Relax, Uncle Z. Grog is boring.'

'Be that as it may, your old uncle has been deliberating extensively.'

'And?'

'You've less than 2 weeks to go, pet. When you finish your commitment a bon-bon awaits. How would you like to accompany me to a medical conference on a popular Caribbean island? I've forgotten which one, but they're interchangeable.'

'Oh, Uncle Z!'

My remaining days of penance dragged by, thankfully without major incident. Last I heard, Jimmy and Fiona Nesbitt were still hitched. He was as happily acerbic as ever. Now that the children were older and he'd some leisure time, Jimmy drank and painted – too much of the former, not enough of the latter. Fiona toured a lot with that warbling group of hers. Doing quite well, she was. I left that island off an island off the island without a backward glance. Petra Neumann was welcome to it. I was sailing off to a different fate.

What had I digested? No point in trading addictions. Endgame in isolation was hideous. I sent a prayer over the waters for the predispositions to dissipate before temptation jumped out of its box – or needle – again.

And another thing: I wanted a man and a different kind of love, one that included stability, not the 'Sleepy Lagoon' sort of arrested development. 'Two people in tune, two hearts on fire' no longer attracted me.

I wanted more.

Pieces of eight from Graham, Joseph, Herman, Ian and Errol ▬▬▬

Wayne Cooperville

'Medicine has deposited waves of confabulators and boors at my feet, and one amazing wife,' said Wayne Cooperville. We nursed margaritas in a decaying seaside bar with flapping wooden shutters. 'Thank you, Graham Greene. Tommy MacDonald and I finished medical school and travelled the country surfing with our first wives. Tommy submerged himself in Joseph Conrad, to feel the wind on his face. I stood alone like the throb of a lighthouse pulsing in the stormy night. I was starting to welcome its dark embrace. Until I met Amaranth and realised that I wanted more.'

I'll leave poetic descriptions of ocean, sky and wind to Tommy MacDonald. He joined the navy to escape hierarchies and competitive medical systems and pander to his wandering genes. The navy shipped him off to God knows where to wreak his own brand of insubordination on unsuspecting senior officers. I inherited his position on the HMAS *Hawke*. After reading *Our Man in Havana*, I was determined to test my sea legs. Naval medicine would form me into a rounded and experienced doctor. Or so I told myself. Not only that, but the mythical creatures of cryptozoology – the study of and search for legendary animals – lured me. Who knew what cryptid might confront me in the Indian Ocean? Wherever my hobby led, I'd decided not to confide in officers or crew.

I didn't care a hoot whether I felt the wind and spray in my face. The engine's vibration and hum were not a nourishing comfort but an admonition to hypervigilance. Out came the medical books, starting with Manson's and nutritional deficiencies. Pellagra – that curable lack of the vitamin B complex – didn't plague people in Central America, possibly because their maize was treated with lime or because they were coffee drinkers and coffee is high in niacin. I wanted to apply some preventive measures, like adding quicklime to the ship's water supply. It might also prevent pellagra, but I didn't trust my epidemiology. That particular vitamin deficiency was more common among stokers than sailors in the eighteenth and nineteenth centuries, as well as any institutionalised group forced into hard, sustained physical labour on a diet poor in fresh fruit, meat and vegetables. We were well stocked with those, and powdered milk and eggs. We weren't big on polished rice, so I'd no expectation that beriberi would cross my path.

My stint in accident and emergency provided much of the experience I was likely to need and gave me confidence to face the unexpected. Knocks on the head and split lips from drunken brawls would account for most of my patients, who would be fit, young and middle-aged men. I'd face none of the ailments afflicting women, children and the elderly. What could be more straightforward? Or so I thought.

A string of uneventful days and nights rocked me into a false calm. Soon I was ready to discharge the public health component of my duties. Or so I thought.

I read navy manuals in transit to the coral atoll Diego Garcia, the southern-most of 52 islands in the Chagos Archipelago midway between Asia and Africa. The United States military wanted it in the 1960s, so the British government obligingly relocated the indigenous Ilois 1000 miles away to Mauritius.

This was new to me. I was merely another recent medical graduate seeking his anchor in the vastness. Navy protocol taught me how to draw fresh water on board for sterilising in a foreign port. Add so much quicklime to the tanks and then pump in water from the barges that bring it out to the ship. Sounded straightforward enough, but no one had yet implemented this procedure as this was the HMAS *Hawke*'s first voyage out of home waters. Our results in Diego Garcia were memorable.

'Where's the quicklime?' I asked the engineer, a sour, misogynistic man with needled hair.

'Dunno, doc,' he replied. 'We'll ferret around.'

'Let me know as soon as you find it,' I said. 'I have to calculate the volume of water we're taking on board and the amount of quicklime we have to add.' The aim was to achieve the appropriate level of chlorine to sterilise the water. I used obscure formulae in the calculations. Next day, the engineer plunked his tray down near me at mess. We sat with some of the crew. It was the weekly pizza night, so the men were happy. 'We've found some old brown paper bags of white powder, doc,' the engineer said. 'Think it's the quicklime.'

My calculations must have been out a little bit.

'Hey doc, what'd you do to the water?' asked Tug Wilson. Tommy MacDonald once nearly misdiagnosed his severe constipation as appendicitis.

'Sterilised it, Tug. Why?'

'It smells like a bloody swimming pool.'

'Tastes like one, too,' chimed in Jim McGuinn, the medic.

Sparkie and Chippie, the electrician and carpenter, voiced their agreement.

'We're in the bloody tropics, doc. What are we supposed to do?'

'We can't drink our tea or our water.'

'Tryin' to poison us, doc?'

So they drank and drank and drank goffa, our Royal Navy's term for soft drinks. I took some ribbing from the troops over my miscalculations. When a lot of them got diarrhoea from eating ashore, they blamed the water and what I'd done to it, so I wore that, too.

Never mind. I'd plenty of time for my hobby. I was reading a new, definitive work on cryptozoology and hung out on deck at appropriate hours for whatever sightings the deep wanted to offer.

Quite early one morning I was up on deck hoping for a sighting when McGuinn the medic ran up. 'I told Radar I'd find you,' he said. 'He's staggering towards sickbay.'

I followed him down to examine the patient, wondering what could be wrong.

At 6 feet 5 inches tall, Radar Chambers was too tall to be a comfortable sailor. He was also cavernously thin, despite possessing the appetite of an ox. Shipboard life for Radar was one continuous round of bumps and lumps and bruises and the development of a permanent stoop as he navigated from bunk to boiler room. He got his nickname because he handled the ship's communications, just as the chief petty officer was called Tug because of his surname: Wilson.

After settling him on the examining table, I asked, 'How long have you been shitting through the eye of a needle, Radar?'

'Since right after you done the water, doc.'

'You ate ashore, right?'

'Yeah.'

'Might've come from that.'

'Naw.'

'How frequent is it?'

'Bad, otherwise I wouldn't be here.' His frown accentuated his close-set eyes. His round cheekbones, riding low on either side of his face, made him look like a startled sea serpent.

'Abdominal pain?'

'Yeah.'

'Nausea?'

'Yeah.'

'Vomiting?'

'Naw, but my head's pounding.'

'Any skin problems?' I was checking the diagnostic triad for pellagra: diarrhoea, dermatitis and dementia.

'Like what?'

'Redness.'

'Nah.'

'Itching.'

'Nah.'

He'd no signs of dermatitis, so I did the standard checks for dementia.

'Who's the queen?'

'You mean Elizabeth?'

'Of course.'

'Thought you mighta been talking 'bout a musician or some poofter.'

'What's the name of this ship?'

'HMAS *Hawke*. Why're you asking me these stupid questions?'

He was too young for age-related memory decline. No dementia.

'Fix me up, doc.' He lowered his voice. 'This is my last trip.'

'How's that?'

'Promise not to tell anyone?'

'I promise.'

'Sure?'

'I've taken an oath.'

'Come closer. It's top secret.'

I leaned in.

'I think I've found buried treasure.'

So began a convoluted tale. He may have been confabulating: spinning stories that sound plausible but are fantastic. A confabulator came into hospital once when I was a resident. His story was too elaborate to have been concocted. I smothered thoughts of what a doctor would conclude during a consultation if I came in babbling about a cryptid sighting.

As for Radar's physical illness, I was adrift in a sea of possible diagnoses. Diarrhoea was obvious. Dermatitis, definitely not. Probably not dementia, but I was fairly inexperienced. Two out of three and it might be niacin deficiency. He didn't appear to be pre-pellagrous. He was far from irritable and morose, his complexion was not muddy or bluish and I spotted no skin lesions. Nor did he complain of a burning sensation in the oesophagus. In those days, *Norovirus* was not a consideration, that saviour beloved of cruise-ship companies to cover a variety of litigious, incompetent diagnoses of conditions from which people generally recover in a few days without long-term health effects. Contaminated shipboard surfaces such as doorknobs were ideal transmitters when many people occupied a relatively confined space. Experts don't consider *Norovirus* to be a risk in an open environment.

As no one else presented complaining of diarrhoea, the probable diagnosis for Radar Chambers was, *Something you ate*. My prescription was fresh meat, fruit and vegetables, and a lot of them. I judged him not to be a danger to others.

'It's something you ate ashore, Radar.' Or drank.

'Or drank, doc, like your water. Once I find my buried treasure, I'll be right.'

Sailing into the dark unknown can cause all sorts of terrifying visions – even on a navy vessel – of strange leaping creatures. Ancient maps and charts warned, *Here there be monsters*. As in Gloucester Bay in 1817, what I sighted out of Diego Garcia was 60 feet long and barrel-shaped with a snake-like head. I was bursting to tell someone, so floated my idea by the captain, who asked what I'd been drinking, suggested a trick of the light and clouds on the water and finally admitted to more things on heaven and earth, Horatio, and especially on the sea. His closed and banging fist punctuated the conversation, which gave me a certain sympathy for Radar Chambers.

Compared to my new vessel, navy ships were well organised with essential medical equipment like the drip chamber I needed for a drunken Englishman. I signed on with the Caribbean cargo ship to test myself professionally and to search different waters for sea creatures, and I'll admit to a certain amount of wanderlust. I'd sailed the Pacific and Indian Oceans and wanted the Atlantic under my belt.

I wasn't yet professionally settled. My first marriage started to break down after we got me through medical school and celebrated our release with a surfing trip round the country with Tommy MacDonald and his first wife. The foam and waves bought us a few years, but when I returned from Diego Garcia, we faced the hard facts and parted amicably. I packed Manson's – just in case – next to Bailey's *Physical Signs* and set sail. I was ready for anything.

I've always been the retiring sort who finds chit-chat a chore. I prefer a good book to a *bon mot* and conversation orchestrated by the private dervishes whirling round our hearts. Graham Greene instilled in me the desire to sail the precise seas that might deposit me at Cap-Haïtien if the winds rebelled in the hurricane belt. It was well before the earthquake, right after 'Papa Doc' Duvalier and his son made Haiti the poorest country in the Western Hemisphere aided by their secret police, Tonton Macoutes, the bogeymen in dark sunglasses. I didn't make it to Haiti that trip, but I got close.

In addition to the crew, I was responsible for seven passengers: two middle-aged couples cruising together who were no bother, two anonymous single men who kept to themselves, a bagpipe-playing Englishman and an elderly lady I called the *grisette*, after those independent, nineteenth-century Parisian working-class girls.

Shipboard, I always preferred silent heroes and adventuresses. People should keep their mouths shut in most social situations. Many spoken words are unutterably banal, especially fuelled by alcohol, earnestness or sanctimony. And now interactive Internet. The poetry of Conrad's prose, the ineffable craft of Greene, the non-whingeing, non-litigious swashbucklers of old: all flounder in the seas of universal access to travel. Now bloggers sue cruise lines for their upset tummies. Our times have made the true adventurers obsolete. Even on that cargo ship, the insipid replaced the intrepid, trivialising life in this age of marketers. Being a writer, or an artist, or even a trained medical practitioner meant something before the masses got their paws on a little bit of knowledge. More democratisation, less magic. The lowest common denominator was woefully ignoble. Cruise-ship marketing quadrupled tourism in 20 years, adding families with toddlers (now, I ask you!), young couples and honeymooners to the wealthy and well-heeled retired. No longer was it a once-in-a-lifetime event.

Gone were the civilised and opportunistic whom Graham Greene encountered on the high seas: the eccentric; the ageing *grande dames* cloaked in sequins shadowed by fortune-hunting young men with pencil moustaches and glinting teeth; the old colonels yearning for battle; wealthy couples whiling away the time; single and silent men, nefarious or anonymous, slipping in and out; and governesses and teachers en route to distant Empire outposts in search of husbands or, failing that, a dignified single life. Standards were maintained, evening clothes worn, manners appropriate and appreciated. Tradition flourished in shipboard names like Empire Casino, Queens Grill and Lions Pub.

That was before my time. Instead, the sea gave me Peter Wicks, a heavy drinker and nasty piece of work. He brought a set of Northumbrian smallpipes from northeast England from which there was no escape. Day and night he serenaded us, until one day the pipes disappeared. A reluctant crew member rescued them from the cold embrace of the deep, but Wicks got the message and no longer subjected us to that howling.

One evening after dinner in the Queens Grill, we all ambled to the Lions Pub, as was our custom. The two couples sat on banquettes at the arched windows. The other passengers appeared and disappeared. The engineer and I represented the ship.

Wicks hawked and spat on the gold-and-brown paisley carpet, missing the spittoon by several inches. If I'd been more experienced, I'd have lectured him on sanitation. 'I was in a mining accident – wolfram it was, in the Lake District – could have been my fault,' he was saying, 'and decided a different kind of life was for me. The company paid me off, the wife wrote me off and I set off to see what the rest of the world had to offer.'

The Geordie possessed one redeeming feature: his friendship with Lily Alice Duffet, a highly skilled, once-respected milliner's assistant and artist's model. She represented the ghostly navy of workers whose jobs were now irrelevant, as perhaps computer peons will be in 50 years. Cargo-ship travel was quite inexpensive in those days, so Mademoiselle Duffet lapped at the shores of her eternity by going from cruise to cruise, immersing herself in gracious times past. I disagreed with the engineer's assessment that she was dotty – that unrepentant misogynist. She'd merely outlived her usefulness and suffered a surfeit of nonessentiality, living proof that a long life wasn't always a blessing. Mlle Lily was well 'tanked up', as my dear wife Amaranth would say. Her men left her well loved. The attraction for Geordie cannot have been the décolletage proudly maintained and displayed or the coquettish air with which this stately woman sailed the decks.

'Might do a different kind of mining,' Wicks continued, downing another gin. 'There's a 30-square-mile area, in international waters not far from here, supposed to have sixteenth- and seventeenth-century shipwrecks. They've already recovered 18 cannons and a bronze peg. I'll hire some divers and sit on deck playing me pipes. Heard they might have some rubies, in case you're looking to invest . . .'

No one was.

We joked that our ship belonged to the bare-bones class and called her the *Expediency.* Nowadays, you can find the on-board surf simulators, movies under the stars and lawns for sports and picnics. Not on our ship. Not one fitting in bar or cabin was anything other than pedestrian; nothing, that is, except the ballroom or, to be precise, that section of the Lions Pub's floor on which people danced. It was a glorious relic from more generous times. Why it was on a cargo ship I've no idea. Six black marble pillars topped by lotus-shaped lamps flanked a round, inlaid wood floor. The area was demarcated by an art deco frieze lowered from the ceiling, which concealed the music system's speakers.

One evening, the Geordie waltzed the *grisette* round to their song, the 1940 'Sleepy Lagoon.' It was the B-side of the later Platters hit, 'Harbor Lights', I learned from a trivia night somewhere. Peter Wicks was one of those cumbersome people who are astonishingly light on their feet. Lily Alice Duffet was timeless in her shimmering ball gown. What they created transcended reality. I watched for a while, and stepped out on deck as Frank Sinatra crooned 'Goodnight, Irene' sometime between 12:30 and 1:30 in the morning, that hour when passengers go missing forever. I forsook snapshots of this dying waterborne world for cryptozoological ruminations of the nineteenth-century golden age of sea serpents. Erratic, bird-like footsteps approached, uneven and light, pulling me back to the present.

'It's Peter, doctor,' gasped Lily Alice. 'Please come *tout de suite.*' She was the only one who brought out a bearable side of the Geordie. I complied with alacrity.

'What's happened?' I asked as we hurried away.

'He's vomited up blood.'

'What colour?'

'Bright red.'

'Much of it?'

'A litre.'

'And he's been drinking.' Statement, not question.

'Yes, doctor, more than usual.'

This was a major, major danger sign that called for emergency measures.

'Where is he?'

'Sickbay.'

By this time, we'd made our way down, and the patient was on the examining table with the engineer standing over him. 'Please leave us now, Miss Duffet,' I asked, turning to the sour-faced misogynist as she wafted through the door.

'I'll need your assistance. Every second counts.'

'Right you are, doc,' the engineer said.

'We'll have to run an IV drip immediately.' I made a horrifying discovery. 'Where's the drip chamber?' I asked.

'What's that?'

'The bit that counts drops,' I said. 'It's vital.'

'Dunno, doc.'

'Find it!'

We hunted desperately for precious minutes. We'd plenty of equipment for neurosurgery, abdominal surgery, even heroic obstetric procedures, but no drip chamber.

'I'll have to improvise one in a hurry,' I said. My next obstacle appeared. I raked over dim memories of how to direct-match blood and call for potential donors. I think I aged 30 years. Happily, Wicks didn't bleed again. Next morning, I read the riot act over him. After importuning me to buy rubies, he promised to behave better for the rest of the voyage. He was a man of his word. Sort of.

If not for Wicks, I'd not have needed a change of scene and would not have met Amaranth. Ah, *la femme*. Tropical islands were superfluous to my needs, with their miles of beaches capped by mountaintop jungles, but I was desperate to retrieve some of the years I'd aged tending the Geordie. I wanted to stretch my legs in the blue coffee mountains of the island that Christopher Columbus used as a family estate. With any luck I'd see the country's national bird, *Trochilus polytmus*, a long-tailed hummingbird called the doctor bird. We docked in the port whence the world's ships carted away 'green gold' until the banana blight of the 1920s. I hiked to a remote town that was the hideout of eighteenth-century runaway slaves, the mountain base from which they raided the sugar plantations below for 50 years until the 800-plus free Africans were granted independence in 1739.

I almost called into a crumbling house on the way back, nestled into a hillside not 15 feet from the water, of grey stone with a maroon-tile roof and creamy phallic pillars stretching to the sea. Had I stopped I'd have met my future wife and uncle-in-law, but the presence of several tourists deterred me. Instead, I proceeded to a charming town with graceful old buildings, cocooned in the knowledge that Ian Fleming and Errol Flynn preceded me. I strolled towards the twinkling lights of the harbour. Night descended. I leaned against a wooden railing and gazed into the water's depths, reluctant to break the mood. A bell sounded close by.

After some time, I heard two people talking not ten feet away. 'Some of the finest deep-sea fishing in the Caribbean,' a wild-looking girl mumbled to a dignified, impeccably attired European man in buttery loafers utterly inappropriate for the surroundings, but thongs for such a personage were unimaginable. 'Fishing? Me? Tomorrow? Amaranth dear, try to remember that your old uncle has certain needs, like the "quiet but rewarding vacation experience" the conference organisers promised. And no, you may not cross the island to the party side.'

His companion ignored him and said to me, 'You were singing 'Harbor Lights', the Platters' version.'

Most original, and from a mirage of the night-time sea. To my shame, I let down Graham, Joseph, Herman, Ian and Errol with my besotted response. 'I was?'

'Whatever the young man was singing is better than "Everything's all right, gonna have me some fun tonight!"' To see the personification of immaculacy spasming like Little Richard impersonating Moby Dick was positively hallucinatory.

'Look, there's Dr Pito.' She pointed a quavering finger at an even shorter Central European male, intense and bristling, craning his neck at the cannons atop the old fort. 'You need to talk to him, don't you, Uncle Zoltan?'

'No. Yes, Amaranth pet, you're quite right,' he said, raising a shrewd eyebrow, 'I do want to question my esteemed colorectal colleague regarding his emergency surgery lecture.'

With the receding purr of expensive footwear, I and my sea feast were alone.

'Look at the moon.' She pointed as the disc scooted behind speeding clouds, rim glowing over their mountainous peaks.

A mist formed. The moon's halo illuminated Amaranth. Her face was silver and her body indigo. Both dissolved at the edges. 'Get a grip, man,' I told myself, 'you've been alone too long.' It was the sea. I'd not permit any other harbour lights to steal her love from me.

Reason failed me entirely.

Hot diplomats and black-booted gazelles ▬

Malcolm Phillips

'Like many younger sons from the dawn of time, I sought my fortune far from home,' said Dr Malcolm Phillips, peeling off his soft faun gloves in a materialistic striptease. 'That my elder brother was a wastrel engaged in the serious business of frittering away [index finger, right hand] the family pile [second finger, right hand] mattered not in the land of primogeniture [ring and little fingers right hand, first and second fingers, left hand]. I swallowed my pride, swore my Hippocratic oath and sallied forth into the unknown. And [gloves lain neatly next to the microphone] here I am.' With modesty appropriate to his exalted position – raised chin and eyebrows, drooping mouth – he surveyed the journalistic cubs and their decrepit colleagues, all gathered for the announcement of his appointment to a prestigious position on the medical board. Only one reporter knew the truth about his 'pile' and he was scudding from his own sharks.

My patients and I have chosen each other wisely – well, mostly. Two cases of miscommunication were no fault of my own. The first was in Scotland, where I diagnosed a patient without sharing a common language. This was one of my most memorable house calls and came late one summer. I'd finished my residency in London and was treading water, considering my options. I envisioned a practice in an exclusive area with what some would call a trophy wife. Let them. Judge me if you will, but I knew what I wanted after being born into a life of heartbreak, and it wasn't more of the same shackled to more of the same.

A working holiday was just the thing, in a location to rub shoulders with the right sort of person. A colleague needed time away from the practice founded by his grandfather, in which his father also practiced before an early death. Alistair planned to sit an exam in Edinburgh. The locum he'd booked cancelled at the last moment, to his frantic dismay. That's how I found myself in a village in the west of Scotland renowned for fine sea and shore fishing. Perhaps I'd pick up a few pointers from experienced fishermen between sessions with undemanding patients. This village boasted Loch View, one of the world's finest hotels for this sort of thing.

The phone rang at 3:00 one morning.

'Doctor, can you come?' asked an agitated Mrs MacDougall Loch View. The village was so full of MacDougalls and MacFarlanes that people were designated by their addresses. Mrs MacDougall Loch View was the manageress of the posh hotel.

'We have a Polish diplomat staying,' she explained. 'He's on his own and obviously extremely ill. We think he has some sort of exotic disease.' The owner of the hotel was a Scottish MP, a foreign service refugee himself, so members of the diplomatic corps often appeared.

I pulled a coat over my pyjamas and grabbed my bag, tripping on the uneven footpath as I hurried through the windy, moonless night. Tufts of loch brine shrouded my eyes. The only signs of life were the muffled buzz and dull pool of lamplight from the hotel. Through the window I saw all the staff huddled close, the comfortable and bitter alliances of cook, maids and assistants momentarily forgotten in the mutual threat.

Mrs MacDougall Loch View met me at the door in a voluminous electric-blue polyester dressing gown. Where she got it, God only knows. *Why* she got it was more to the point. It hinted at intriguing habits. I was impressionable, unprepared for the variety of night-time attire that would greet me through the years. Worth a monograph, that is. The light bulb overhead etched the facial lines of the anxious manageress. 'This way, doctor.' She trudged up wooden stairs whose sagging middle was masked by a faded blue Oriental runner, echoing the material encircling her own midriff. Her sketch of an ill diplomat sent us on different trains of thought, she of strange deaths caused by bad management and ultimate dismissal, I of a career among the great and the grand. I rejoiced that this opportunity presented itself so early in my professional life and wished my preparations for this important consultation were sartorially appropriate.

As I followed her down a long passageway, I recalled knowledge gleaned from lessons about exotic diseases in medical school. Not much.

'In here, doctor,' she whispered, letting me into a room overlooking the loch, furnished sparsely but handsomely with wardrobe, washstand, table and chair. And a four-poster bed.

All the lights were on. Here was one light switch for which I would not have to fumble. After the receding dimness of a sound night's sleep and the poorly lit corridor, the glare stopped me in my tracks.

'Please, doctor.' Mrs MacDougall Loch View conveyed a tortured plea in those two words. She was my first patient in this stern village and expounded on the threat posed by young upstarts. I felt her plight keenly as she led me to my patient. Dying guests were bad for business, as were those who contracted exotic diseases, and she wasn't getting any younger.

'I'll take it from here, Mrs MacDougall.'

She withdrew reluctantly.

Propped up in bed was a slender man of indeterminate middle age. Perspiration glued lashings of fine brown hair to his broad skull, intensifying the look on his face. He was terrified. He claimed illegitimate descent, I found out later, from the great composer Chopin. He must surely have inherited his nose from that alleged ancestor, and a long, thin, shapely thing it was. At the moment, it was red and dripping, not at all the suave, dignified proboscis one expected on a diplomatic face descended from musical romanticism.

We soon established that he spoke no English and I no Polish. We'd no other language in common in which I could ease the poor man's distress. I'd never been good at languages, and my French was rudimentary. I dropped my black bag next to the bed and pantomimed sitting on the bed and taking his pulse.

He nodded sweaty assent.

His pulse was fine. I grimaced and gazed into the middle distance as if deep in productive cogitation. I was playing for time, hoping something would come to me. Finally, I made eye contact and inclined my head reassuringly to Mr Chopin. This gesture relieved him.

Now what? I withdrew a sphygmomanometer from my bag. Something was wrong. I felt hot, with a faint buzz under my bum.

Of course!

I had it. I laughed and pointed at the blanket. Mr Chopin hadn't a clue what I was doing. Heaven knows what he foresaw. I pawed at the blanket and mimed wiping perspiration from my brow.

His eyes widened with fear, saying eloquently that doctors in Scotland were crazy. Why else would they gesticulate at blankets and shake invisible perspiration from their brows in a hotel room at 3:00 in the morning?

Clearly, I was not conveying my message. Dramatic training in medical school would not be ill placed.

I got down on my hands and knees. He cowered, petrified into inaction. As I slithered behind the head of his bed, the poor patient leapt out and streaked to the wardrobe, which was near the door.

I hoped that the apprehensive Mrs MacDougall Loch View would not invade the intimacy of a doctor–patient consultation. 'Ah!' I cried finally. I looked across at the poor man wedged wide-eyed in the small space between the wardrobe and the wall. A doctor on his hands and knees crawling behind the bed was not a sight to instil confidence in a patient.

Twisting and stretching, I found what I was looking for. I beckoned Mr Chopin.

The diplomat remained immobile.

I gestured again.

No movement.

I glared at him commandingly.

He obeyed, floating towards me as if facing a firing squad. His eyes bespoke impending execution as his hair unplastered itself from his forehead. He was cooling down. When he got close enough, I tugged him by his quivering, clammy hand onto all fours. Mr Chopin must have fancied that his enemies had run him to ground in a bizarre foreign land. I pointed to the wall and to the blanket. I made him touch the blanket's heating coils. Mrs MacDougall Loch View left the electric blanket on, which was new to the diplomat. Simple as that. Nothing else was wrong with him.

Next morning, I was just sitting down to kippers and eggs. One window framed the loch, the other the sea. Clouds chased each other across a gloomy sky. The day's water palette threatened to remain gun-metal grey with ivory foam. Mr Chopin's face appeared at the sea window. He'd come round to thank me. Another round of sign language ensued, this time with eyes expressing gratitude rather than fear. I later received a formal thank you – and payment – from his embassy.

It was a successful home visit. We communicated without words, to the ultimate satisfaction of all. I encased the embassy's letter in glass and wood, and it hangs still on my diploma wall.

As for Mrs MacDougall Loch View, she united her staff, no small feat anywhere but an especial accomplishment in a Scottish village. The last I heard, her position was too firmly entrenched for any bona fide exotic disease to topple her. That chore devolved upon the Grim Reaper, and he'd have a fight on his hands with that determined Scotswoman in her electric-blue night attire.

My second case of miscommunication with a patient occurred in England when I was called to the bedside of a fully dressed unconscious young lady in black leather boots. What do you *do* when such a vision does not respond to any of your requests? She was unable to provide the slightest clue about what had felled her. All I knew was that a young male voice rang through to the surgery one afternoon to say she'd been taken ill very suddenly. He'd promptly hung up without leaving his name or any details other than an address. Serious illness that comes on suddenly is not common, but when it happens it's a disaster if things don't fall right. Quite obviously, she had a temperature, but I couldn't stick a thermometer down her throat. My only clues were the few tiny spots on her exposed collarbone.

The call to this empty house came early in my medical career in this country. The favour paid off, the one I'd done for my Scottish colleague. He passed his exams in Edinburgh with flying colours. Thanks to him, after 2 years in London I'd soon be off to Australia and a partnership in one of the best practices in the land.

A different *terra incognita* faced me that day, a *terra nullius* with not a soul in sight. The room was dim, the lighting poor. I daren't waste time groping for a light switch. I put my hand round her neck, pulling her into a sitting position to remove enough clothing to determine what was going on. She came up stiff as a board. I immediately suspected meningitis. I'd never come across meningococcal meningitis with spots and a stiff neck.

I grabbed the telephone and dialled. While awaiting the ambulance, I observed my patient. Black boots encased long, slim legs. Her skirt and blouse were speckled fawn and white, the colour of field mushrooms. Her neck, I now realised, was long enough to accommodate the entire length of my hand. I'd a gazelle before me. Even in unconsciousness, she looked graceful. This was the sort of patient I wanted. I knew she'd be properly appreciative and no bother. I'd wanted to be a hospital administrator because that leads to real money and I wouldn't have to bother about keeping people onside, but I got a scholarship to study medicine. It turned out to be a good thing. I like the respect it brings.

The ambulance arrived smartly and took my sylph to our local hospital. I followed and whipped upstairs to the clinical library, to better inform myself than the up-to-date doctors in casualty. A quick read informed me that the spots did not resemble anything in the books.

I scoured my mind for details from the youthful caller who'd requested the house call. 'She was well this morning when she went out shopping, except for a sore throat. When she came home, she complained of a headache.'

I left the library and walked down to casualty, through recently upgraded corridors of healing. Gone were the old wood and warm lighting that bespoke a certain sort of doctoring, replaced by the latest offerings of the modern age.

The registrar shuffled some papers in response to my query. 'Undine Pacot. We're going to discharge her.' His rumpled, nerdy look got my back up. We're leaders of the community and have certain standards to maintain. People looked up to us. How could we encourage tidy habits in our patients if our own toilette was slipshod?

'Oh no, you're not!' said I, starting down the hall.

'We'll give her some penicillin,' said he, eyebrows a picture of condescension.

'Penicillin isn't all that young lady needs,' I retorted. 'Start a drip immediately.'

The registrar followed as I hurried to the patient.

Undine was conscious, barely. 'They woke me up, patted me on the head and said it was tonsillitis,' she whispered.

'How do you feel?' I asked.

'Terrible,' she whispered, eyes filling with tears. 'If I'd known I was this sick, I'd have gone to the doctor. James and I were going to the ballet to celebrate our 1-year anniversary, to see *Les Sylphides*, my favourite.' With that, she slid back into unconsciousness.

'She's not going anywhere,' I said to the registrar who was close on my heels.

I crossed my arms in front of my chest and planted myself on her bed. 'If you release her, I promise that every sort of mayhem will visit you.'

That caused a reasonable ruction.

'I want a lumbar puncture on her,' I insisted.

'Hmph,' snorted the registrar.

Fortunately, I was impervious to all the sparks thrown off by his diamond-like brilliance. You'd think GPs would become accustomed to being pooh-hoohed promptly and utterly, as is the wont of so many casualty departments who are dead certain that the local family doctor is a lower form of life – universal phenomenon, occurs in all countries.

I assessed the situation and took the wisest approach. 'I'll pull the general superintendent away from his golf.'

That achieved the necessary.

'Okay,' agreed the registrar reluctantly. 'We'll do a lumbar puncture.'

It presented pure pus. Panic prevailed. 'If she has meningitis,' said one courageous nurse, 'I'm leaving.' 'You can't force me to stay, either,' said a stout-hearted intern. 'She might infect all of us.' They were afraid for themselves, not the patient. Nothing like grace under pressure.

I left, unnoticed by the staff, galvanised into action by self-interest.

I rang up the next day. 'How is Undine Pacot, the young lady admitted for meningitis?'

'Still unconscious, and actually, she has developed rather a nasty rash.'

The young lady in black leather boots recovered, I am pleased to say, and is now a valued member of the community, I hear. That she survived is pure chance. She owes her life to an anonymous phone call and a certain congruence of circumstances.

Whoople the cadger

Dexter Veriform

'My patients have offered me so much, some of it edible, some unpalatable, all treasured,' Dexter Veriform said. 'It started way back on the west coast of Scotland, before we sailed for the Antipodes. I tried to be worthy of that sacred trust between doctor and patient, a bond which no third party has the right to tear asunder, and it has brought me to this prison hospital bed.' He pawed the bedsheets. 'Dr Shipton was never sued. He murdered hundreds of patients after lunch. You're not sued if people like you, and you're much more effective. I'm fed up with being politically correct. Now I'm going to say what I really think. What else can they do to me? They've taken it all, my calling, my reputation, my livelihood, most of my friends and two of my four children – all except Olive and my memories. And the gift of hatred.

Never has doctor detested patient more. Whoople the Cadger . . . even lifting that faraway rock under which he resides sets my teeth on edge. In all my years of seeing patients – and I will call them patients, not clients, to my dying day; my God, I'm not selling encyclopaedias door to door – I can only recall one man whom I disliked as intensely as I do the profession's self-appointed watchdogs. I've lived long enough to observe the nature of hospital administrators change from helpful to obsequious to obstructive to omnipotent.

We GPs are in a vulnerable position. Our life's work can be dismantled by the chip on a wimp's shoulder or the burden in a spinster's heart. Those bureaucrats excel at manipulating others. Male or female, traditional bureaucrats or modern femocrats, they all act the same, and they do it under the government's protective mantle. We GPs are powerless. Aren't we? My darling wife Olive tells me I've begun to rant. Can't be helped. So much is wrong with our profession, and none of it involves transparency, accountability or regulation. I agree it's about power and trust, but whose?

I tend to get on with people most of the time aside from the occasional bureaucrat, but I couldn't *stand* Mr Whoople. Everything he did irritated the *hell* out of me. For instance, he worked at the Forestry Commission and lasted only 3 weeks. It wasn't suitable work for him. Road building, fence mending, caring for young trees, looking after forests, the tree nursery and brushing trees were not for Mr Whoople. *Really*. The Forestry told him not to bother coming back, and he was unemployed again. That suited him down to the ground. Despite being a consummate cadger, Mr Whoople was an entrepreneur, I'll give him that. He rode the bus 14 miles to the nearest town with one or the other of these dames and returned laden with foodstuffs, which he sold round the houses at a tidy profit. He didn't have a car, but Mr Whoople had two houses, and that on the unemployment.

He had two wives as well, who were sisters. Their babies looked exactly like him. He was around 30 and inclined to stoutness, with rusty, dull-red hair and bleached skin. He radiated self-satisfaction from narrow brown eyes that also showed shrewdness and greed. The sister to whom he was not married received a single mother's pension. The sisters thought he was cleverness incarnate. He was what in Scotland is called a nyaff, a miserable little runt who obviously has some hidden reserve.

One of the benefits of working in an over-doctored area is that those patients you don't like can be persuaded to find a better doctor round the corner. The West Highlands of Scotland many years ago was hardly over-doctored. Its denizens were respectful and trusting and none too well off. The difference between year-round residents and summering Glaswegians was quite remarkable. No local called me out frivolously. The Glaswegians were *much* more demanding, always wanting me to come to the house for quite trivial things. They irritated me, but we made a lot of extra money from them because they were temporary residents. We were paid by the government to manage them for the year.

The Forestry Commission brought people like Brian Whoople from Glasgow, for instance, and provided furnished houses on its estates and bicycles for workers to use for work. It also built, all over the west, neat little rows of two- and three-roomed wooden cottages. They were like little villages consisting of 30 or 40 houses.

I was at the clinic one day, seeing out one of my favourite patients. Mr Gillespie was one of the stable West Highlanders who worked on the land or in the forests. He lived with his wife and bairns in one of the two or three forestry villages in the district. Nobody touched him for mending fences. He took such a pride in his fences that I wondered if he'd named all the posts. 'Tell the missus I'll be out later,' I said. The good woman had recently delivered her third child.

I whistled happily until I saw the three lumps of human flesh sprawled across six chairs in the waiting room. One poor oldie huddled in a corner with her knitting and overcoat. The set of her mouth showed the stories backing up behind it, waiting to disgorge into afternoon-tea tales.

I'd no choice but to nudge all three lumps towards the consulting room, where Mr Whoople presided during the antenatal examinations. He talked continuously and interfered.

'You're disrupting the consultation,' I repeated. 'Please go to the waiting room.'

'Oh, Brian, stay,' the sisters insisted.

Finally, I realised I was engaged in an exercise in futility. They were the sort who would accuse me of doing something naughty to them, for the money. 'Keep quiet, Mr Whoople,' I ordered.

He was awful, simply awful.

'How are you feeling?' I asked Sister A as I took her blood pressure.

'She's a'right,' Mr Whoople answered.

'Please let her speak for herself,' I said, with uncontrolled asperity.

'I'm a'right,' Sister A mumbled, head down, stringy blonde hair falling forward. Both sisters inherited pale-blue eyes set so far apart they appeared piscine. I wrote her blood pressure down on her card.

'Can you feel the baby moving?' I asked, preparing to listen for the heartbeat.

'Can we feel it moving?' he said. 'It's a regular little squirmer.'

'Mr Whoople, please,' I said sternly.

'Yeah, it kicks a lot,' said Sister A.

'Excellent,' I said. I checked the baby's heartbeat and turned to the other sister. 'And you, dear?'

'She's been off her food,' Mr Whoople said.

'Mr Whoople,' I said warningly.

'Wha'?'

'Keep quiet.'

'I'm a'right,' she said.

'No, you're not. Give her something, doc.'

'Your appetite okay?' I asked.

'Whaddya mean?'

'Are you off your food?' I asked, using his phraseology. Sister B might be depressed. I particularly wanted to talk to her alone.

At this point in the examination, the father-to-be turned to Sister A and said, 'I'm thinkin' we'll get some sugar and onions to bring back and sell.'

'I can carry the onions,' Sister B said.

I knew Sister B was the younger sister and felt she needed to prove herself. I desperately wanted to talk to her about her marriage, but dare not raise anything sensitive with that arsehole hovering round. I felt frustrated in the extreme at the total emotional block he created. It wasn't the general lack of respect that bothered me – that was nothing new – but the altered dynamics of a relationship that to me was sacred, the inhibition of both parties . . . and a self-preserving intuition warned me about being sued. Thank God I didn't know then that Mr Whoople's ghost would hound me to this day.

'I'm a'right,' Sister B stoutly insisted.

'No, you ain't,' Mr Whoople said.

'Yes, I am.'

'Stop arguing, woman! Dexter, I want you to give her something.'

'It'd be better for the baby not to, *Mister* Whoople.'

'I've heard of this new wonder drug, tal, thal –'

'Thalidomide. No, it's too untested.'

'My women deserve the best. It's a wonder drug.'

'We don't know that.'

I didn't prescribe thalidomide for either of those sisters, thank God.

I once actually bought a reel-to-reel tape recorder – not a compact one like nowadays – and recorded an interview with one of these dames. It's astonishing how much he interfered with the examination. For credence, I recorded it. In Britain, they don't have the same training system as they have here. A trainee is allocated to a trainer for a year. He actually becomes part of the practice. I played this tape to mine. He said, 'You've got a real cheek recording that without his permission.' My request would have been refused. Of course it wasn't fair, but he might have acted mannerly and I couldn't have that artifice. He was an *awful* fellow.

You should think very, very, very carefully before you create an embryo. A lot of babies are conceived in the backs of automobiles. The girl must be in tip-top condition. So should the sperm. We might snag a few more tip-top people. Specimens like Brian Whoople reproduce themselves like mad, but thoughtful, intelligent genes are not replicated as readily.

Luckily, Whoople and his women weren't long in the area. I heard that Sister B delivered a healthy baby girl who looked just like her father.

The UK's National Health Service stretched before me in all its constricting wonder. The freedom of the Antipodes beckoned. Olive and I found ourselves bound for New Zealand and our ultimate destination, Australia.

Forty years of dust and spit

Barker Kaye

I plucked out a tiny insect that was flailing in my Thermos coffee. I'd not long returned from South India and experienced my usual re-entry problems, at least until I found my arboreal paradise in the Tasmanian rainforest. Asian coffee and tea plantations with mist-ringed upper reaches had nothing on the chirps, croaks and creeks on my land. Where else would I hear this tearing as I ripped the bark from freshly fallen trunks and peeled it back in whippy strips 10 or 15 feet long? The hollow of a tree trunk when I thumped it with the butt of an axe differed from the muffled whacking of an unbarked, newly cut tree. Wattlebirds squawked overhead, shrikes trilled and cockatoos cawed. Flies buzzed. Wind rippled eucalyptus leaves.

Four o'clock in the afternoon, the flat hour of longing and remembering, longing for what lay around the corner, recalling the four o'clocks of my past, the loco-motion of patients who puffed and wheezed and who with their maladies drove me to this train in South India at four o'clock in the afternoon.

Four o'clock in the afternoon in third class near Bangalore unleashed cavern-ous visions dappled with shadows and light that morphed medical practice in the suburbs into a straight line to hell.

Four o'clock in the afternoon unfettered heat so devilish that my bones felt transparent and dust gritted my lids, silvering the sheen on life's familiar objects, like the backpack around which one sticky leg hooked.

Four o'clock in the afternoon, the time of Mrs B, who taught me that few actions lack the opportunity for regret. Yes I'd disentangled from the glue of suburban obligations, but she caused a twinge, that patient who needed me most. Mrs B, lovely old dear, always wore the same hand-knitted, multicoloured cardigan buttoned tight across her chest. Mrs B, a tea lady in her day, gently coughed what I feared was pulmonary tuberculosis onto cream biscuits and sugar as she wheeled her trolley from office to office, floor to floor. This journey was partly for her. Or so I told us all, including you, old friend. I feel guilty that I gave notice, that I let you down after your dewy-eyed panegyric on comrades and isolation. I said it again and again: lung diseases and their awful suffering provided my original motivation for entering medicine, when chronic obstructive airways disease carried away my gasping grandfather.

Four o'clock in the afternoon has its own rhythmic clickety-clack, full of wonders like the sea of stunted men in short-sleeved shirts that surrounded me. They dictated that every window in the carriage not jammed in place be wrenched wide open. I was the only Westerner. I stood out like a jumping salmon in a tin of torpid sardines. I licked dust every time I moistened my pearling lips, not the red dust of Nigeria or the Australian outback but the bleached flutterings of a parched land. I shifted positions and left a littoral of sweaty dirt on the narrow bench. Sir John Crofton's comment niggled whenever someone hawked and spit on the floor. Tuberculosis may have come from an organism in the dirt of the primeval muck.

The train swayed through the heat of four o'clock in the afternoon. I scratched dust from my elbow to exorcise the heat-drenched human noise, not with one lone fingernail but a battalion of eager fingers. My mind clickety-clacked between two grooves: sleep and deep questioning of the relevance of medical academics to those of us at the coalface.

The train carried me closer to a remote Tibetan settlement in South India, where another wonder awaited me: Blackmon, my medical academic friend, burrowed within its monastery, immersed in the religion of an exotic culture. He'd lived among Tibetans for 5 years and spoke the language well. The residents in his settlement desperately needed medical attention. Our mutual experience, me as doctor and him as translator, inspired Blackmon to enter medical school later as a mature student. He settled into academia and participated in the Millennium Ecosystem Assessment, a global group of hand-picked academics whose 5-year commission was to evoke possible future scenarios. My curly-haired friend is an expert on the effects of global ecosystem change on human well-being, but that's another story. For now, I wasn't interested in new conceptual frameworks for tuberculosis. What could I do when multiple drug-resistant tuberculosis presented at the coalface? That was my brief.

It was four o'clock in the afternoon and I was seeing patients, not in the 'burbs but in the camps. Blackmon translated, unruffled by the weight of the maroon-and-saffron monk's robes that engulfed him. The heat of the day liquefied one o'clock, two o'clock and three o'clock into a thousand iridescent droplets which snaked down my neck and coiled in the small of my back. We'd done a home visit that morning to a shack in which Granny coddled her two-year-old progeny. The house was dark, with only one tiny window set high up in the wall, and the bedding never aired, Blackmon determined. Tubercular Granny coughed solicitously upon her beloved.

I shifted on the wooden chair, my haunches squelching and melting. The concrete floor of the consultation room embraced the edges of my feet. Laminated posters on the walls displayed cascading bodily systems and functions. One small window welcomed the breeze, such as it was. Periodically, light fractured into beams that split Blackmon's shoulders into a thousand atoms.

I cleared a handkerchief-sized square on the crowded desk, refraining from claiming too much space out of respect for the usual doctors. I leaned back. An ominous creak shot me upright faster than I'd moved all day.

'Right, Blackmon, shall we call in the next patient?' I said. Clearing my throat might retrieve certain dignities.

I liked him immediately, as soon as he stepped through the portal, that awful tubercular hack preceding him. He sat on the edge of the chair facing me. One look at Tenpa Dawa at four o'clock in the afternoon told me much of what I needed to know. I forgot the heat and my discomfort as the consultation deepened. My patient wore that badge of success, Western jeans, along with a pink polyester short-sleeved shirt purchased in healthier days. He seemed to be disappearing within his clothes. Soon, only his eyes would remain, huge and bewildered, a caricature of the dreams of man.

I looked at his notes. Tenpa Dawa was sputum-positive when discharged from a 6-month stay in a sanatorium a few hundred miles away. I cobbled together the rest of his history with the aid of my valiant friend. Tenpa spoke street English, but I preferred Blackmon's nuances for our purposes.

'How old are you?'

'Late twenties.' He looked far older. Tibetans were casual about age at the best of times. Escaping in mortal fear over the Himalayas through a whitened world of pelting snow was not conducive to the transport of official documents. They didn't have birth certificates anyway. Our customs were not theirs.

Visualising snow instantly soothed me. Maybe Blackmon was practicing some similar sort of cooling mind control.

'Do you have shortness of breath?' I asked.

Tenpa nodded, his coarse black hair already flecked with grey.

No need to ask about a cough, not after that hack announcing his entrance.

'Night sweats?'

Blackmon conveyed this question with physical acrobatics.

No, no night sweats. I flagged this item with an explanatory asterisk. Through the paneless window a bold scarlet blossom lifted her head in the barest breeze. Nowadays, in an increasingly globalised world, treating patients without a common language is not as problematic.

I listened to Tenpa's chest and percussed each lobe, observing his general condition. He was thin and wasted, as tubercular patients tend to be, but did not have cachexia, the extreme wasting that appears before death.

I reached for Tenpa's right hand and examined his fingernails. They'd not yet become the little clubs evident in advanced lung disease, including TB and cancer.

'Have you been taking your medication?'

We sorted out what and for how long and when he'd stopped. Like many Tibetan refugees with tuberculosis who attended our clinic, Tenpa did not understand 'compliance.' I've no idea how Blackmon conveyed the concept. Patients got better after a while and stopped taking their medicine. We in the West acted the same with antibiotics. Who were we to talk, particularly when a course of the only treatment available could run for 18 months, like TB medication? 'I was feelin' better, doc, so I left off taking the last few tablets.' How many times have I heard that?

'Are you working?'

'He's a sweater seller,' Blackmon translated.

Itinerant merchants called sweater sellers were the worst defaulters in that settlement in the south of India, on land given by Nehru to Tibetans fleeing the

Chinese invasion of their homeland. Tibetans travelled from city to city, laying out their goods on dusty, polluted sidewalks. They lived in appalling peripatetic conditions and saw different doctors in different cities for medication, when they remembered. Sweater sellers were often away 6 months of the year – long enough to disrupt any course of treatment for tuberculosis. A poem came to mind I'd read on the train.

> I am tired
> I am tired selling sweaters on the roadside,
> 40 years of sitting in dust and spit.[4]

'I'd like to spend more time with you, Tenpa, but 80 patients are waiting.'

He smiled and said in English, 'Okay okay, doctor. I am tired anyway.'

'I'll be here for the next week if you need me. Anytime.'

'Thank you, doctor.'

I couldn't do anything for him. 'Blackmon, can you please explain to Tenpa that he needs to stop spitting, if he does. And tell him why.'

I wouldn't tell him to stop kissing, like one older colleague who worked in an English sanatorium in the 1950s which discouraged mouth-to-mouth contact and forbade open-mouth French kissing. You probably wouldn't contract tuberculosis from saliva, although it was possible. No point in making him a leper. At least his TB was probably not too virulent, but it would be highly resistant.

What's the solution? I treated tubercular patients for a few days in that settlement, but so what? Conditions were desperate. Dormitories were dark and overcrowded with monks fleeing oppression. Their beds were so tightly packed they actually touched. Bedding was never aired in the abundant sunlight. I toured sickbay, where conditions were exactly the same. One poor monk was coughing copiously, without covering his mouth. This was 20 years ago. I hope things have changed, but last I heard tuberculosis remains one of the most intractable problems threatening the health of that exiled community.

It's the same problem my friend Tommy MacDonald faces when working with Aboriginal communities. He doesn't want to move to Australia's Red Centre permanently, but what good are a few scattered weeks? He's now got three GPs with whom he alternates 6-week stints. That wasn't practical in this case. I held clinics for a week and wandered round India for a while, trying to process it all. Blackmon returned to the West and applied for medical school. We met again some years later, at a conference whose keynote speaker was a brilliant researcher specialising in the effects of global ecosystem change on human well-being. But as I said, that's another story.

Other four o'clocks crisscrossed at different velocities. At four o'clock in the morning, I deplaned in a Delhi dream and joined a wave of dazed Westerners in an exit queue. The ceaseless round of snuffles and funny turns receded, a car zooming in the opposite direction that also carried an elephant of a passenger: my impending marriage. The press of bodies funnelled me past a stamp-wielding official to an impenetrable clot of auto-rickshaw drivers. The noise, the noise, submerged the West in my heart. Men shouted unaccustomed rhythms into the

---

4 Tsundue 2007.

unquiet night and spewed atonal music at top volume. Car horns honked in short blasts and prolonged wails. I didn't care. I was in India! My mind morphed from lancet to sponge.

At four o'clock in the afternoon, I perused a dinner invitation from a drug rep over a cup of tea while waiting for a software program to open on the computer. I never could resist a generous feed, whatever the attached strings. I was enmeshed in suburban general practice, working for a friend who was taking his first break since medical school. By chance, I sat within conversational distance of Zoltan Nagy across an expanse of starched white linen at a generously sized table. Quite the raconteur he was, expounding upon his early days in medicine. Zoltan wielded a butter knife for emphasis as he recalled the numerous admissions of an alcoholic patient to the Royal Rubicon, the state's only mental hospital. He was quite fond of the man, as he was of all his patients, or most of them. This alcoholic came into the surgery one day with a cough, worried he'd picked up something nasty from the tea lady, who wheeled the tea trolley through the several floors of the business, coughing gently all the while and spreading what he feared was tuberculosis. Between bouts of drinking, this man worked his way up from errand boy to president of the company. Zoltan knew him in his prime and tended him on the long slide back down. I listened in a desultory fashion, pondering how thickly to slather butter on my roll. I was young, with loads of time before my arteries would harden. Zoltan's words halted my knife in midair, on its way back from the butter dish. 'Did the tea lady have pulmonary tuberculosis?' I asked. 'Almost certainly.' He stared at my butter knife. 'And your patient?' I drew the yellow wedge onto the plate. 'No, luckily for us.'

And for me. Drug companies be thanked.

The lassitude of one Sunday afternoon at four o'clock enchained me. I was explaining to my fiancée why I needed to bolt. I protected the many reasons too sacred to send out as cannon fodder in the male–female wars, clustered around *raison d'être* and The Big Picture; and mumbled about being a tinker, not a cottage cat like Thomas MacDonagh's 'John-John,' who set out at six o'clock in the afternoon. Once again, I pierced the heart of my love, and hated myself. But I needed my secrets. Still do.

Regarding India, I'd told something different to my patient Mrs B, my betrothed and my boss, all parts that didn't shape a whole. Even now, all these years later, when conditions of heat and dust and longing conspire, Tenpa Dawa coalesces into an iridescent taunting spectre and I scratch my elbows and still, still, the fragments don't add up.

But I keep looking, at four o'clock in the afternoon.

'About the size of a ▬▬ potato, doctor'

Petra Neumann

Dear Pieter, [she wrote] Only 15 years, not much over aeons, but enough to extinguish a way of life by such niggles as the way we're communicating now. *Blasted server. How can it be down again? I'll unplug the connection and plug it in again . . . there!* To continue our conversation begun at the Antwerp conference last week: you asked me why I'd left my son with his father and gone to the city. It was the boy's choice. He was 10 years old when I left – 15 now – and so firmly rooted in that remote community, with its family networks and traditional ways, as to be inextricable without permanent damage. We're close, though: as much as we can be through email and annual visits. He's happy, truly and deeply, so I know I've done the right thing. Let the jealous and tiny-minded corrode others with their verbal acid of 'unnatural' and 'bad mothering.' When you know in your heart something's right, it can require more courage to loosen certain bonds than to tighten them to strangulation. Here's how it happened, since you asked.

I knew my days in urban practice were numbered after Mr Dean came looking for me with a gun upon his second release from the psychiatric hospital. I chose the remotest spot I could find, an island off an island off an island, a greasy little dot on a small splattering from a big splash. I loved the city, but always harboured a needle of wanderlust, a need to push boundaries. Vagabondage ran deep in my family. I imbibed it with mother's milk. Every year during my childhood, the family went walkabout for 4 months in an old caravan, bookending summer. My parents always extricated me from school, I've no idea how.

A forgotten corner of the earth offered an antidote to a schizophrenic patient wielding a gun, convinced I'd ruined his life and determined to impose justice. Somewhere like the Anonaka Islands. A ferry off a boat off an airship. Huge great cliffs cast sheets of shadows far into big seas. Near the wind-blown edge of whitecaps and rubble huddled a rare patch of green, two stunted acres of trees in a sea of rock. The prevailing wind sheared the treetops flat, bequeathing a bleak beauty.

Only 33 of the hundreds of islands were inhabited. Many were single-family islands whose only outside contacts were the visiting doctor and teacher and the boat that picked up wool and dropped off stores twice a year.

Remote locations present an extreme against which we city and suburban types can test ourselves. They attract what André Soubiran called freaks, outcasts and outlaws, only he was talking about a leper in a Paris slum.[5] What awaited me in a faraway land? It turned out to be the same old thing. People went about the business of living and dying, keeping warm and fed and loved. I joined in, singing my version of the same old song. But I'm galloping ahead of myself.

To me, the Anonakas were an adventure, the logical extension of my childhood ramblings, the next stage in the life of one unwilling to tread the wheel of time like a manic rat trapped in the spokes. These noble notions trotted through the bright day. The real truth whispered in the dark that I was a spooked mare on the run from a patient. *Can't get away fast enough from Mr Dean and his dangerous delusions, can you, coward?* galloped after me through the night. Easy for me to romanticise this remote location, but the islanders were trapped, resident by fate or design. Those silent, stoic, self-sufficient folk were prepared for anything, except perhaps a lady doctor with progressive ideas.

Here I was in my early 30s, wearing trousers which they all found peculiar, dishing out condoms which they all loved. For them, abstinence started with doing the right thing, which included dressing appropriately to meet the new lady doctor.

Only a couple of women appeared at my first outlying clinic, come to check me out. No men came at all. None, except one old man, with trouble sleeping and blocked waterworks.

'Only the one,' I related later to Charles, my senior partner.

The early part of my time on the islands was spent with such other jetsam – as we foreigners ironically referred to ourselves – as Charles, Jimmy and Fiona. My senior partner's many many years in the navy had left him with a taste for grog denied during his youthful missionary days. Absence from land developed a crust round the old sea dog that made him unwilling to discuss his early life, except when liquor cracked the armour and the words oozed. At odd moments, when no one was looking, Charles' expression assumed a cast-adrift countenance, not so much far away as loosed from its moorings in threatening waters. Undertows, rip tides: words for a man who patiently kept watch on the bridge between twilight and dawn, as Soubiran says.[6]

Charles laughed. 'They expected me, so they wore their normal work gear.'

'So what?' Back home, people came in wearing any old thing.

'This is their first experience with a female doctor, so of course they all went home.'

Two thousand people lived in the islands. They perpetuated an odd mixture of old-fashioned ideas and expedient practices I found shocking. Back home, we'd have been arrested for some of the things they did, like polyandry. Women were in short supply, so it was not unusual for them to be married seven or eight times. If things were really looking bad, they moved on to somebody else. They

---

5 Soubiran 1954. p. 175.
6 Ibid. p. 83.

changed partners, but they always got married. That was socially acceptable behaviour; a consultation with the new lady doctor in your work clothes was not.

The next week found Charles laughing again. 'We told them you were coming, Petra, so all the men turned up in their suits and their shirts and their thises and their thats, and they were absolutely furious because they got me!'

After that, the men realised they never were going to know who was coming, so it all sorted itself out.

This demureness and respect extended to following doctors' orders unquestioningly, like practicing total abstinence for birth control, which resulted from Charles' religious ideation. No wonder people were demented when I arrived. They'd no contraception at all, no Pill, no condoms, no rhythm method. I could not work out why my first few patients were off their trolley. A house call on a sick child provided the answer.

One day, the radiotelephone rang at the clinic. Could I come out? Little Pearlie had a fever. As sometimes happens, the child was the pretext, not the patient. The child was fine. I left the cold bedroom for the warm kitchen and a cup of tea with the parents. Mr McShane stoked the peat fire. He turned at my entrance, the flames jumping in his spectacles. He wore his wife's Dame Edna glasses ('I found them in her drawer, doctor, and they're the only ones I can see with'). It was not uncommon in the islands for men to pull out these diamante glasses, men rippling with muscles, in dungarees and checked shirts, like Mr McShane, with grease on their hands from working with oil and sheep. Their lack of vanity was quite amazing, especially when combined with their insistence on sartorial correctness.

Mr McShane blurted out, 'This is getting pretty hard, doc. How long does it have to go on for? We've already done it for a year and we don't think we can do it any longer.'

'Do what, Mr McShane?'

'The wife'll tell you,' he said, stoking the fire to cover his embarrassment. 'Mother!' he yelled.

Mrs McShane strode in, all beefy farm wife. 'He means *relations*, doctor,' she whispered.

'Relations? You mean sexual intercourse?'

He nodded, stoking the fire furiously.

'One *year*?' I was incredulous, not because they'd gone without for that long but because they'd followed Charles' antisocial advice so completely. I wish my patients nowadays were that compliant.

'Yes, doctor.'

'And other couples?'

'The same.'

'Leave it with me,' I said, a plan already forming.

Three weeks later, a shipment arrived from the International Planned Parenthood Federation. The only problem was that 24 *crates* of condoms arrived instead of the 24 boxes I thought I ordered. So masses of packing cases of condoms, with 12 boxes each, were piled in the corridor, in the tea room and wherever else was necessary.

A surprise awaited us. One box per crate contained coloured, multifaceted, extravagant inducements to safe sex. The rest were ordinary. Matron confiscated the interesting boxes because they were not really *nice*. 'Maybe we can tolerate plain condoms, just,' she told me severely, 'but coloured condoms are not |bang desk] to be had [bang desk] in the colony [bang desk]!' We never knew what she did with them.

The condoms worked splendidly. Charles was quite put out.

'You can say what you like,' I told him, one morning between patients, 'but this is how I practice, and that's it.'

With his partner and his patients so adamant, Charles couldn't fight it.

Not long afterwards, Mrs McShane called in with a jar of her beautiful tea-berry jam – made from an indigenous, metre-high shrub with little red berries – for helping her out of a jam, she said. I still think of it.

My first 18 months passed in a blur. I took up horseback riding, from necessity rather than pleasure. I stayed off boats when possible and avoided assignations with large sailing vessels.

The condoms calmed the islanders, but they were no less reticent. Their provision made me popular, fortunately, as I hadn't the foggiest idea what I was doing in the radio clinics. It was years before the fear subsided that I'd be unmasked as a fraud. The whole islands always tuned in to find out who'd got what – 10:00–11:00 every morning – on the same frequency, so it got pretty tricky for doctor and patient.

Today, numerous telemedical services exist. Maritime radio-medical services such as one funded by the Italian government provide medical assistance to doc-torless ships. Others offer similar assistance to Swedish and Danish mariners. On land are the Singapore General Hospital and the Royal Flying Doctor Service in Australia, that lifeline to the bush. Our system was different, our patients impass-ive. No instructing anxious mothers to give their babies one teaspoon of Bottle 17 from the refrigerator regularly for so many days; no, nothing so straightforward.

One morning, I sat down at the wireless, which was on a table. Someone had considerately faced my chair towards the garden. I appreciated that, but soon forgot even the cup of tea at my elbow. I set the clinic in motion with a twirl of a knob and some apprehension. I was at that phase of my career when I would say to patients, 'Hmmm, that's interesting, I think I just heard the phone.' I'd dash into the other room and frantically look it up in the book. 'Gaawww! I wonder what that is! It looks a bit like this.' I would rush back. Even simple things like plantar warts can be quite daunting if you've never seen them. Nowadays I say to patients, 'Hmmm, I don't know what that is. Let's have a look in the book,' especially for dermatology and such.

A young woman's voice crackled on the airwaves. 'It's Victoria here, doctor.'

'Oh yeah? Victoria, how are you?' Sip of tea.

'Wellll, same problem as before.'

'When was that, exactly?' I asked, madly trying to place Victoria.

'This would be right after you got here.'

'Ummm, can you give me a clue?'

'No, but you'll know. It's the same problem from a year and a half ago.'

I was working blind, knowing that everyone in the islands was listening. Someone would guess if I asked Victoria for general hints about troublesome body parts, so I tried to remember who she was and in which settlement she lived and work it out. We worked without notes, because you never knew who was going to ring. I actually got quite good at eliciting a history and working out what was wrong without giving too much away. You start with 'How are you feeling?' and go from there.

Finally, I said, 'Ah! Would it be the time I came out to you?'

'Yep! That's it.'

Victoria had a vaginal discharge.

'Got it. I'll send you something out.' Sip of cooler tea.

'Fine.'

I worded it so she knew what was happening. I could always write a note.

'Something else, doctor.'

'Yeah?'

'I've got a lump in my groin.'

'Yeah?'

'I can't come in because my husband is away sailing and the kids are at home and they're only small. It's quite painful.'

'How big is the lump?'

'Well, you know, sort of like a lump sort of lump.'

'Well, how big's that? Is it like' – nobody knew what a golf ball was – 'a big fist or a small fist?'

'Oh well, um, it's not big, I suppose.' Size was relative.

'Is it tender or sore?'

'Sort of, sometimes, I suppose, but it's really sore when I pull up the bucket from the well.'

It was hard days for women in the outlying settlements. They drew water and carried it for miles to their houses.

'Are you feeling unwell with it?'

'Well, no, not really, just tired. No, no, I'm all right. When will you be out here?'

'Not for another 3 weeks.'

'Oh. Well, I'll see how I go.'

The next morning, she rang back.

'Um, this lump's bigger.'

'What size is it now?'

'It would be like a potato.'

'A big potato or . . .'

'No, a little potato, but it'll be about like a potato.'

'Where exactly is it?'

'Well, it's sort of on the line where your pants are.'

'Is it tender?'

'It's really, really sore now when I draw the water up from the well.'

It sounded like appendix, or perhaps a hernia.

On the third morning, Victoria said, 'You know, I don't feel so well now. This lump, it's sort of like a medium-sized potato now.'

It was growing too fast for a tumour.

'Look, you're going to have to come in. This is silly.' Sip of cold tea.

I sent Jimmy to bring in Victoria. He made a face and ordered me to announce over the airwaves, 'Fiona Nesbitt, if you're listening,' I knew she was, she'd never miss this, 'Jimmy will be late for dinner. We need him to pick up Victoria.'

When she staggered in, Victoria showed me a huge lump the size of a large grapefruit. Removing her clothes revealed a mass sitting in her right iliac fossa, which she interpreted as the size of a small potato sitting on her groin that really, really hurt when she drew the water up from the well, but otherwise was not so bad.

Mining families ▬▬▬

David Snow

I like to go for drives round here, look at the moonscape. We're mostly hard-rock mining, like tin and copper. Soft-rock mining, as for coal, is dirty and danger-ous and has gas. Firedamp, ignited by shot firing, contraband or coal dust, or propagated by coal dust, was a major cause of mining accidents in England and Wales. AJ Cronin's doctor stories told the tale. The ground here is stable and less likely to collapse. Families are tough, but they pay a price.

Fishing is far more hazardous than mining. All these drowning deaths because the weather's so rough: as well as you know the weather, you can still get caught. On the other hand, miners sustain more injuries than fishermen, and some pretty bizarre ones. Like the Tawsons. Three of their five sons sacrificed body parts, and one contributed the whole noodle.

The gambling addiction of the eldest Tawson boy landed him in gaol regularly for fraud. He befriended middle-aged widows with that lost look of his and embezzled their lifeblood. Last I heard, he was back inside. The second son got away, moved to the mainland and was never heard from again. The rest of them stayed here. Number Three met the worst fate, Number Four's quick reflexes saved his life and Number Five was the most interesting of all.

A while back, the hydro was building the power station out at the dam. Roundabout dawn one day, the phone rang. Could I come out and certify Johnny Tawson? The old lady's third son was driving a dozer and had misjudged a rock. The impact threw him out of the cab. The dozer rolled over him and cut him in half. They pulled his body partway out from the machine. I squirmed underneath to declare him dead. Cresting the ridge afterwards revealed clouds sailing across the valley. I remember the beautiful drive better than the hapless miner.

Mining is less labour-intensive than in the past. They use great big machines rather than hand-held drills, so when accidents happen usually two or three guys aren't hurt unless it's an accident with a truck or a freak collapse like in Beaconsfield, in northeastern Tasmania. Out here, they don't do the old-style mining and there is very little hand-held drilling, which is done by gun miners who use drills at face height. They're usually not big men. Being 6 feet 4 inches tall in the old mines meant hitting your head all the time or always knocking your limbs on something. The ideal was short and stocky – strong and nuggety. Older miners with experience were best. The ones who stayed the course without going back on the dole tended to finish up in their early 50s, when they got sick of it or wore out physically. It's nowhere near as physical now, although they do lug drill bits. They all use machines, so they're sitting in front of a control panel.

Agility was important, that and fast reflexes, as old Mrs Tawson's fourth boy, Will, found out. He was working a bogger underground one day. By that, I mean a centre-articulated mining vehicle that looks like a front-end loader. Will's job was to dump the ore from the stope into a truck, which would haul it to the surface. Unfortunately, a design fault nearly ended Will's life. One day he was removing ore from the stope and stood up in the seat. He had to peer over the side to know where he was going. He reversed, and for some reason the bogger stopped and threw him off. That machine rolled on and squashed him between itself and the rock face. 'It just kept coming at me, doc,' was how he put it later. Will crawled away despite a pneumothorax, a collapsed lung. The other miners extricated him and brought him up to the hospital. X-rays showed he'd broken his collarbone. He'd sustained cuts and various abdominal injuries. 'You're lucky, Will,' I said as I stuck in a chest tube.

'The family luck must be changin', doc,' he whispered. He still works here as a mechanic part-time, but not in the mines.

Number Five Tawson added restlessness to the family tradition of being frowned upon by the gods, an unfortunate combination given their bad judgement. Young Jake attempted a bit of this and a bit of that in the mines, and was always discontented. He should have followed his second-eldest brother into the world before settling down to look after his mother, but these men never do. It was common: youngest child as sacrificial carer. It wasn't always a smooth fit. Sometimes, they were temperamentally unsuited to the job – and it was a lot of work.

His discontent spilled over into his love life. Young Jake couldn't keep a girlfriend. He spun from one to the other to the next. Before long, he'd exhausted the entire supply of women in these parts, young and older. One day, he informed his mother that he was taking a bride, a Filipina lass. Quite a few of them lived among us. They were lovely girls. Who could blame them for wanting a better life? Mrs Tawson nearly expired on the spot, which would have suited everybody; instead, she lived on – and on – to greet her new daughter-in-law. To general surprise, the women got on better than did husband and wife or mother and son. Jake was happy to go to the mines and work the conveyor belt.

One night, the phone rang.

'Can you come out right away, doc?'

'What's happened?'

'It's Jake Tawson, doc. He's caught up in the conveyor belt. We need to get him out.'

I threw on my jacket, grabbed my black bag and rushed straight out into the cold. I played all sorts of scenarios involving various states of mangled flesh.

One of the men was waiting for me by the lift. We were soon rattling downward, deep underground. I strapped a miner's torch round my head and soon arrived at Jake's side. They'd pulled him out. I switched the torch on and knelt by the injured man. He was conscious, barely.

'There was a rock on the belt, doc,' he whispered. Like most miners, he was clean-shaven. Weren't many beards around, though miners might not shave for a few days because they couldn't be bothered.

'He used that thing to take it off,' said his mate, flicking his hand to indicate the steel pole with which Jake dislodged a rock from the continuously moving belt. You have to stretch for the emergency lever to turn off the conveyor belt.

It took only moments to determine that he'd broken his arm badly, in three places.

'It pulled his arm in,' his mate explained. His head followed.

'Good thing you were wearing your helmet,' I said. 'It's the only thing that saved you.'

'What'd you say, doc?'

No wonder he couldn't hear: his helmet was squashed down to half its normal size and had rubbed off his ear. Later, someone in the city fashioned him a new ear, one of those artificial ones you clip on. Convenient during spousal spats.

The accident left him with burns to the hand of his unbroken arm that later required skin grafts. At one stage, we contemplated amputating Jake's arm. He kept that, and it prevented his return to his old job when he went back to work. He was lucky not to be killed. To Jake, his family lived under a cursed star, and that was that.

I run into Jake sometimes, and he remains miserable with his lot in life. Unlike his wife, who's as nice as can be. She looks after him uncomplainingly, and her mother-in-law. Jake ended up being the most fortunate of all the Tawson boys, except perhaps Son Number Two, the one who got away.

The Tawsons were one kind of mining family. There were others, like the Gaskins and the Armstrongs. The intersection of those two was quite a story.

Never lend a patient money or anything else. An involuntary smile may cross the features of those of us simpatico with drug addicts, alcoholics and gamblers. I haven't always acted in my own financial self-interest. It wasn't any of the above or an abandoned young mum who bested me, but circumstances and plain justice in the form of Curly Gaskin during a consultation.

Not all mine managers were hard-hearted paper-pushers who worked their men to the bone to maximise profits for the company. Plenty of those slithered around under rocks, don't get me wrong. I hated doing health checks on their men because they pressured me to certify all the workers fit. Enter Curly Gaskin. His great-grandfather came out from the north of England to run a mine on the mainland goldfields in the late 1800s. He hated the heat and brought his family down here. His son and grandson, Curly's father, managed the big tin mine over in the northeast. As a boy, Curly loved to watch the big pumps suck it up from hundreds of feet below. They blew away a lot of basalt over its top, which was done on a large scale. The process mesmerised the boy.

Curly knew from the beginning that he wanted to live around mines. Not underground, no, at least as little as possible. His father would not have allowed him to become a gun trucker – or mechanic – or a gun miner working a drill at face height. Nor would he have allowed his son to be a storeman, ordering equipment and supplies. Becoming a doctor and working in a mining town was a possibility, but his maths and science scores were weak. A process of elimination led him to follow in the old man's footsteps. It took me years to smoke out this much, chipping away at his rocky reserve patiently, in the surgery, at the football club and at endless summer barbeques. The rest I gleaned from other townspeople.

Gaskin even looked like a miner: short and powerfully built. He'd long ago lost his coppery hair and eyebrows. At 35, he was balder than the pub's billiard balls. They called him Curly. The mining company executives told us to call him Mr Gaskin. Charles. Charlie. He hated Charlie. They said 'Curly' didn't project the proper image for their company. Once again, they demonstrated how out of touch they were. Curly treasured his nickname, telling the bosses it was crucial to the issue of respect, but they continued to call him Charlie in a tone of false bonhomie which he despised. Their consistent unyieldingness was a sign of things to come.

Lawless Armstrong also entered the family business, like those generations of coal miners in Wales. His ancestor was transported from the north of England around 1850. He'd worked the seas and done something heinous on land in a bout of drunken bad behaviour. Out here he worked as a piner for years, first as a convict and later as a free man. Lawless bored us with tales of this man living in a badger box, a wooden inverted V construction overlaid with bark and thatch. He felled massive pines, barked them, sawed them into required lengths and rafted them down the river. His son, Lawless' great-grandfather, worked a different facet of the same alluvial flats when tin was discovered in 1891. He wrested it from gravel beds with a pick and shovel. He despised the isolation and inclement weather, and having only the wildlife for company – echidnas and lizards, snakes, wombats and wallabies, gulls and ravens and currawongs – he worked in a tin mine and lived with all the other miners in a big hut made of galvanised iron. Photographs from the Boer War plastered the walls. Their two-tier bunks lined one side, topped by bag mattresses stuffed with straw. They cooked in a big fireplace at one end of the hut, baked bread in camp ovens and ate tinned bully beef, bacon and dried peas. Lawless' great-grandfather planted a garden of peas, potatoes, carrots and rhubarb. His grandfather and father also worked the tin mines.

Lawless was proud that his family history was the same as the area's: first whalers, then sealers, piners, prospectors and miners. We'd all been cornered in the pub and shown a tattered photograph of an Armstrong in flannel shirt, thick-soled hobnail boots and felt hat peaked in the front.

Lawless' one goal in life was to join the 25-year club, with its annual meeting established by the mine for workers who'd put in the long hours. These days it's rare to spend that long in one place, let alone in an itinerant industry with less job certainty, what with contractors. Bit like shearing, I suppose. No one would be eligible for that club nowadays. Even if you started with one company, you'd go elsewhere or go on the dole, ready to chuck it all for unemployment benefits. Not Lawless. He was determined.

I knew it. The mine manager knew it. Everyone knew it. Except the bosses.

Lawless Armstrong got his nickname because he did everything by the book. It drove us crazy. We all knew he'd never lie. He wanted only to go back down the mine and harangue his mates for each minor infraction of the rules. He couldn't do much lifting anymore, so the question was, what to do with him? Lawless' general health, as that of his mates, was tied to the lack of diversity of food, tobacco smoking, alcohol: lifestyle and the mining culture rather than the work per se, as people faced in many remote areas. He smoked and drank a lot of beer, but that lessened with 12-hour shifts. On traditional 8 a.m.–4 p.m. shifts, he'd stop off at the pub on the way home. With 7 a.m.–7 p.m. shifts he and his mates went straight home. Rosters these days depend on the mining company and can be 8 days on and 6 off, 7 days on and 7 off, 2 weeks on and 1 off or 1 month on and 1 month off.

Curly Gaskin's family defended a long tradition on the other side of the fence. He traced his people back to the 1500s, or at least his surname, which was derived from Gascoigne. His wife scoffed, but he insisted they name the children Henry and Isobel, after his sixteenth-century ancestors.

By the time the Armstrong and Gaskin families intersected, a culture of fear and intimidation was rapping at mining industry doors. We were going backwards with new industrial laws. The guys were told, 'Sign here now or get out.' Pay decreased to $100 000 per annum over a 10-year period because somebody else could do the work. Wages rose when a labour shortage came along. Miners are the best-paid workers in the country, because the work is dirty and can be dangerous. They can earn $90 000 a year with no experience at all. The average salary is about $150 000 a year. Top miners earn a lot more.

That the bosses called the manager Charlie and the men called him Curly encapsulated his dilemma: divided loyalties. We all knew where Curly's loyalties lay, and I think the company suspected. That he did what was right confirmed their suspicions when Lawless Armstrong tumbled. It was not a bizarre injury like those afflicting the Tawson boys, but it was debilitating nonetheless and made him completely unfit for mine work, in my opinion and in Curly's. The bosses disagreed. A long battle ensued. Curly knew it would be costly and tried to save the company the expense of court costs and legal fees. They weren't interested. To them, Lawless was malingering. Both Curly and I insisted that Armstrong was a good worker who wouldn't file a claim unless no other way existed. But the company's two accountants appeared – a woman and an Indian from South Africa, both with something to prove – and that was that.

So when Curly came in that day for the first time in years, I listened attentively.

'Feels like I've got birds in my chest, Dr Snow,' he said in his matter-of-fact way. Indicating my stethoscope, he said, 'You'll probably find it's a bit wonky.'

He was right. Cardiac arrhythmia. I did the usual history and examination, and ultimately an electrocardiogram. I didn't think he needed a Holter monitor, but I wanted to be sure. When did he first notice it? What were the precipitating and alleviating factors? I took a family history and enquired about frequency and duration. I knew he wasn't an alcoholic, but checked anyway. No, no vomiting, and he wasn't dehydrated.

'I'm sending you to a cardiologist in the city, Curly.'

'I'm not going. It's not so bad. It comes and goes.'

'You must. It could happen at any time. Do you want to be driving and kill yourself and your passengers, or other people on the road?'

'If you insist.'

'What's bothering you, Curly?'

'Lawless keeps after me,' Curly said. 'He's only 26 months away from the 25-year club, and he begged me not to turf him out. The bosses don't want him out, either. But you and I know the truth.'

'It's not right to keep him on,' I said.

He nodded his bald head. 'You know what a stickler he is for the letter of the law. I've appealed to his sense of justice and begged that he show me a way to keep him on.'

What do you do with a guy who tumbles off a piece of equipment and fractures his scapula, his shoulder blade, a few ribs and one of his lumbar vertebrae?

'What can I do, doc? He didn't work out as storeman or back underground. He hated counting bombs.'

Detonators, with ammonium nitrate. They all have to be accounted for before they fire. There are set times to fire, like the end of shift. They can't fire during. They might have loaded up 6 hours before end of shift, but all fired at the same time.

'He can't lift anything heavy,' Curly continued, 'so we can't do much with him. His back hurts too much to do what he was doing before.'

I swivelled in my chair, which made Curly smile, a welcome sight.

'That means you're thinking, doc.'

'That I am, Curly. How can we make it worth his while to leave?'

'That'd take some doing.'

'But it's possible.'

'A big payout.'

Often in the end, injured workers got paid out. The negotiations dragged on, often for years. The general payout was $700 000 – not a lot for the rest of your life after you became self-employed.

'Yes, and fighting for it might mean my job, and Henry and Isobel are teenagers now.'

I grunted in heartfelt commiseration at the breathtaking expensiveness of adolescents. My years of keeping the financial fires stoked loomed in an endless procession before me. I'd never be able to retire. I pushed that spectre away.

'And what if the mine closes?'

'Those rumours I've heard . . .' All the men were stressed about losing their jobs, so Curly's actions were particularly courageous.

'Yeah, doc. Something needs to be done for Lawless, and soon. I want to do right by him, and if it's the last thing I do with this outfit, all the better.'

I leaned forward.

Curly mirrored my movements.

'What does Lawless want most?' I asked.

'To join the 25-year club.'

'And what do we want for him?'

'To be taken care of for the rest of his life.'

'I may know of a way to obtain both the payout and club membership.'

We lowered our voices and hatched a plot, a secret between us and the local lawyer, who gave us a huge discount but needed to cover expenses. I'd my objectivity and wallet to protect (it wouldn't do for the doctor to be considered a soft touch) and Curly wanted to keep his job. We pledged top secrecy about our negotiated payout plan.

One night, my wife was especially nice to me. I was suspicious, and asked what she wanted from me. We'd been married too long for illusions. She got huffy, and said only that she approved of what I was doing for Mr Armstrong, like all the women in the town. I groaned.

We viewed it as a loan, hoping that Lawless would reimburse us from his big payout. We'd have done it anyway, but didn't want that noised about. I won't bore you with the years and tears of legal battles. Anyone who's been through it knows how it changes one's perception of human nature. Our case was different in two respects. First, we wanted to drag it out and delay signing whatever documents the solicitor shoved at us until the last possible moment so that Lawless could achieve his goal. Once it was all over, Lawless' employment would be officially terminated. Second, both the bosses and Lawless wanted him to stay on. They didn't prize his long-term health, and Lawless wanted to pile up the hours. It was an odd situation, to say the least.

Meanwhile, the company kept Lawless Armstrong on, doing this and that; at the end of the day, no one was quite sure what, but it made everybody happy.

As I've said elsewhere, mining companies no longer view themselves as social-service organisations. They tell us to get used to the idea that we're a town with mining in it, not a mining town, you know that sort of glib crap. No, we don't. Bloody economic rationalists. Can't wait for the pendulum to swing back. Hope I'm around when it happens.

One day, I got a call to go down to the mine. Curly had fainted.

I was soon jumping those metal-mesh stairs into the prefab block. A secretary led me into Curly's office, her face creased uneasily. Lawless bent over as much as his back would allow, eyeballing Curly on the floor.

The injured miner struggled to straighten up, using the desk's corner to brace himself. 'I don't usually have that effect on people.'

I'd been keeping a quiet eye on Curly whenever we met, watching for cardiac arrhythmia. I asked Lawless and the secretary to leave us. As soon as we were alone, I knelt down and asked, 'Are you taking your medication, Curly?'

He shook his head.

This might be the first presentation of epilepsy, which in an adult meant a brain tumour. There was one exception.

'Ever have a head injury, Curly?'

'No, doctor.' He was alert, exhibiting none of that ictal confusion, that vagueness experienced by epileptics for half an hour after a fit.

I straightened my back and stretched my neck, avoiding the obligatory girlie calendar pinned next to a genealogy chart. Various door slammings had loosened the pins over time, so the good-time girls gazed seductively from the wall at skewed angles.

'You've worried yourself into a right state, Curly. Are you exercising?'

'You know I hate football, Dr Snow.'

'I insist you start taking your tablets. Don't want to lose you, not yet.'

'I was feeling better so I cut back. I hate taking the things.'

'You need to check with me before you do that.'

'A few butterflies have been fluttering round recently.' He indicated his chest region.

'I want to see you regularly in the surgery.'

'Keeping an eye on me, eh doctor?'

'Too right I am, at least until this business with Lawless is over.' The mine manager took things to heart, literally.

The mine did indeed close down a few years later, but not before Lawless got a nice little payout. I think the fact that he squeaked into the 25-year club meant more than that seven-figure sum we won him. You can guess where he spends his days.

Curly got a job nearby. The zinc works snapped him up. He's still not taking his tablets like he's supposed to.

And yes, in the end we got our money back.

Knives and old lace ▄▄▄▄

Nicky Doulton-Brown

I turned on the SUV's air conditioner, trusting that my dear daughter's batteries retained enough juice to handle it. I was never one for physical discomfort. Why put up with what we don't have to? Speaking of discomfort, one of my wives – I've forgotten which of the four – once asked me to please have a word with the patients who called me out frivolously. That was asking a lot. A yellow streak in me admonished, *Thou shalt not offend.* I lumped it and my wives bore the brunt. They resented my performance. I raised a hell of a noise, like some drug addicts, and like Mrs Thomas with her knives.

Speaking of neighbourhoods, twice I converged with the police and the ambulance on the same street, within Mrs Dymphna O'Reilly's orbit. The two ex-military men and their families still formed an island of law and order at the upper end. The bottom remained no-man's-land, but not for long. Time passed, and gentrification was almost complete. The antisocial behaviour caused by drinking had disappeared. Almost.

I was sitting down to a steak one night, just cutting into a beautiful piece of meat when the telephone jangled.

'Can you come quickly, doctor?' Mrs O'Reilly asked. 'Mrs Thomas is acting strangely.'

Wilfreda Thomas was in her late 60s, with just enough money to be a secret drinker. My wife ran into her regularly on the high street, the expression on her simian countenance sometimes rosy and beaming, often sallow and scowling. Mrs Thomas always dressed in bright yellow – an unfortunate choice, considering her colouring and build. She was, as they say, broad across the beam – so wide, in fact, that she resembled the cross upon which Our Lord was crucified. She was like my wife at the time, sacrificed on the cross of marriage. Her husband had worked in a factory and consumed large amounts of beer. Broken dreams and barley hops claimed him some years back. She rewrote the story of his demise to fit the occasion.

This widow liked her vodka. I didn't pester her much, because her husband beat her regularly and the children had scattered. She was all alone.

Now, the family always owned a series of dogs of all sizes, which never lasted long. On my most recent visit, she displayed a black Scottie terrier – the mother of our little treasure now eying his chance to demolish my steak.

'What is Mrs Thomas doing, Mrs O'Reilly?'

'She's on her doorstep with an Alsatian and a meat axe and won't let anyone in. She's been throwing things and carrying on, so I called the police and the ambulance.'

The police have the power to apprehend people who are a danger to themselves or to the public, but a lady with a knife and a large Alsatian is not a police matter.

'What did the policeman say?'

'He wanted her to go back in the house. She told him to get stuffed. He said to ring you. He's outside now.'

End of steak.

My wife was silent as usual, but the atmosphere thickened. With dire admonitions to the dog, I departed to charm a large canine and a lady with a cleaver who'd imbibed too much vodka.

The Mental Health Act was different in those days. You took along a policeman and an ambulance officer if you made an order to commit somebody. The latter were only allowed to handle people who'd been subdued and were lying flat. They wouldn't touch anybody who required holding down. Guess who settled things down? The local doctor.

I concentrated on my first problem as I drove the city streets: how to deal with the Alsatian. He was a big fellow. Now, I get on with dogs. The average one won't bite you if you tickle him under the ear, pat him on the back and tell him he's a good dog, unless he's trained to savage anything that comes in the door. But if you're frightened of dogs, even a chihuahua will bite. One partner was eaten by all the dogs in the district. He couldn't stand dogs, and they reciprocated. He wouldn't go on a call unless the pet of the house was locked up, no matter what its size. He regularly got his trousers torn, and ended up divorced as well.

I pulled into the driveway and jumped out of the car. I'd devised a plan. Big dogs love to chase cats. It's their one aim in life. If you shout, 'Cats!' or whisper 'Catsssss' and his ears go up, you've got him. I decided to give it a try.

'Cats!' I shouted on the way to the doorstep.

The Alsatian's ears perked up.

'Catssss!' I whispered in my most sibilant voice. That did it. Off he shot, seeking felines in the back yard.

I approached the missus. 'Come on,' I coaxed. 'You're upsetting all those gentlemen down here, and the neighbours. Give it to me.' A cleaver might hack a nice hole in you if you got too close.

Mrs Thomas hesitated. She was pissed off her rocker. She'd been on the vodka for some time. 'Uh,' she grunted finally, slowly holding out the nasty-looking weapon.

I took it. 'Let's go to the bedroom so we can give you something to help you relax.' I hustled her into a horizontal position for the ambulance man to whisk her off.

'But doctor,' she mumbled several times before we got her into bed and on her back.

'There's something for you in my bag, Mrs Thomas.' I turned away for a syringe of sodium ambutol to knock her out. 'Now then.'

I turned back.

I froze.

She'd got a paring knife.

I put down the syringe on the bedside table. 'This won't do, my dear.' I persuaded her to part with it.

I rummaged for my syringe, turning my back on her once more in all innocence.

I faced her.

I froze again.

She'd got another cleaver!

'Give it here,' I said sternly. 'This *really* will not do.' I had an anxious moment until she reluctantly released that axe. I was no fool. 'Let's have a look under that pillow, Mrs Thomas.'

'But doctor.'

'I'm afraid we'll have to.'

'But doctor,' she repeated in her cracked voice.

'Come, come.'

Reluctantly she allowed me to lift a corner of her pillow. A veritable armoury of kitchen knives flashed under all that lace.

'But doctor.'

'You're safe now,' I assured her. 'I'm here to look after you and the police are outside to protect you. Here's a little something so you can sleep.'

And that was that. The ambulance man took her off to the mental hospital and the psychiatric people.

Basically, Mrs Thomas exhibited not so much madness as antisocial behaviour. It is behaviour that the neighbours cope with until eventually it goes too far. You don't see this much nowadays, at least not in my area. The population has changed. Drinking habits have changed enormously. People have benders and go off silly, but they don't drink as steadily or in as great quantities as in the old days. Nowadays, you can't drink as much because you can't drive a car if you do.

By the time I got home that night, my nice piece of meat had lost the blush of youth and required our sharpest steak knife to negotiate. My poor wife tried to hide her exasperation. She'd kindly protected my dinner from the terrier, who met me barking at the door. He knew where I was headed and dogged my every step. I was glad to have him close. I faced the danger of being cut by a larger blade than a steak knife or all of Mrs Thomas' knives combined: my wife lashed out verbally with some real rippers, but nothing antisocial.

I converged with the police and the ambulance on that street another time. We were called out a lot for domestic violence in the 1970s – lethal when combined with alcohol.

'It's him, doctor,' whispered the ever-vigilant, long-suffering Mrs O'Reilly. 'He must be on something, or drinking.' She referred to her neighbour, Shep Skurley.

'Let the poor man live his life in peace.'

'But doctor, he's chopping up the furniture with those samurai swords of his.'

'How do you know, Mrs O'Reilly?'

'Listen.'

I strained my ears. Nothing.

'Can't you hear that?'

'No.'

'Must be something wrong with your hearing, doctor.'

'Mrs O'Reilly . . .'

'Listen! Can't you hear those splintering sounds through my bedroom window?'

'All right,' I said. She wouldn't give up until she'd got me out. 'I'll be right over.'

I slammed down the receiver and started for the door, grabbing my black bag.

'Oh no, you don't.' My normally compliant wife blocked the door.

I blinked.

'We both know that young man has a hot temper, especially when he's been drinking.'

She was right.

'I refuse to let you go out alone.'

My wife spoke. I obeyed. I dropped my bag and rang the police. 'We have a guy with a samurai sword who's going to do some terrible damage.'

A huge sergeant and a constable arrived as I pulled up to the Skurley house. 'Ambulance man is on his way, doc,' the sergeant said. We filed past the rubber swans, rusted cars and bullet-pocked gnomes. Inside, I tripped over a bicycle toppled in the wake of the police ahead of me, who strode down the coffin-like passageway to the kitchen and living area at the back.

'Let me go in first,' I called. 'The sight of you two may incense him.'

'We're happy with that,' the sergeant said, turning, 'but we'll be right behind you.'

One look told me I'd been wrong about the drink. Bad drugs was more like it. Not prescription drugs like his hero, Elvis, but something which made him paranoid, aggressive and dangerous.

Sure enough, Shep was hacking at the kitchen table as we entered, the one at which his mother-in-law always served sticky pastries and sludgy coffee. That redoubtable woman and her daughter Thalia, Shep's wife, stood quivering near the stove. His brother-in-law was nowhere to be found.

'Shep,' I ventured, approaching the rock star but staying out of weapon range.

'Oh, it's you, doc.' His kiss curl wobbled on his forehead, exaggerating his Elvis sneer. 'Remember I mentioned *iaido* that time you came out because of Thalia's cramps? It means "the way of mental presence and immediate reaction." Advanced practitioners use a sharpened sword, not an unsharpened *iaito*, with a t.' He raised a large sword over his shoulder, both fists gripping the handle, and thwacked it down on another part of the table.

'Put it down, Shep,' I said, taking another step forward. 'I'd like you to tell me what's on your mind.'

The police were silent nearby, ready to intercede.

'Well, guess what,' he said, ignoring my request. 'I've graduated. Who wants to use a poncy *shinai* like in kendo, which doesn't even teach drawing and resheathing techniques? I want a stiff sword, not a flexible one.' He spotted the police and said, 'What'd you bring them for?'

'So no one gets hurt,' I said.

Up flew his arms. And down. 'Smooth and controlled, controlled and smooth,' he said, 'and wham! Whop and bam! Oh so coolly remove the opponent's blood from the blade and replace it in the *saya*, the scabbard.'

'Shep, what have you taken?'

'Only some pills, doc, that somebody told me prevent the Big C. And besides, it's her fault.' He swung the sword at his wife.

The police stepped forward.

'Shep,' I warned.

'I love the smell of the *same* – that's the stingray-skin handle, pronounced "sahmay" – after my sweat builds up.'

All that was left of the table now were the four legs. The man of the house swiped so grandly, sword parallel to the floor, that he decapitated two legs at once.

I stepped over shattered coffee cups whose contents pooled on the linoleum floor. 'Time to stop chopping the furniture into kindling, Shep,' I said.

'Gotta keep doin' more to keep the fans happy, that was why I first switched from kendo to *iaido*. And now I can't go back. It'd be like using one of the kitchen knives of old Mrs Thomas down the street, or the kukri her husband brought back from Nepal.'

The sergeant, with the authority of size, and I with that of my profession persuaded Shep to put down his sword in a traditional Japanese way, on a little rug on the floor at the base of his display cabinet, whose doors were flung wide open. The police took him away at half past midnight. It made the newspapers, and sales of his latest recording skyrocketed.

He and Thalia separated shortly afterwards. Just as well. Her people never did approve of him. She remarried a family friend and was deliriously happy, last I heard. Her GP, one of my partners, says she's no tidier at home. The rock star decamped to plague another woman with his four obsessions of cancer, samurai swords, tyre swans and Elvis Presley. I heard he fathered a baby by a groupie. He sold the house at a tidy profit to an upstanding young couple with a toddler and an infant, leaving Mrs O'Reilly immersed in neighbourly tweeness, yearning for more interesting times.

Whitefella dreaming 2

Tommy MacDonald

> The camel boy disappeared into the desert. The man with the cross gave our mob good water and strange food and made them sing about his spirit god. It was okay. The rock holes were empty. Maybe his spirit god talks to theirs and the water comes.

Delirium claimed me the night I ran into a tree to avoid hitting a camel. Or shock. Or visions. I dragged myself out of the Toyota and kept warm by moving my limbs. At first light, an old Ford rattled down the track and got me out. Broken ribs, broken leg and some other nasties keep me housebound now, back in the 'burbs, finally able to dabble in painting.

The spirit of Eddie Mayfield glides my paintbrush across the canvas. My ancestors demand the swirling texture of oils. Watercolouring is not for a land of little liquid where Dreamtimes throb, where time is not the linear foe of our acquaintance. I'm aiming to snare that concept in this painting, a representation of the base clinic in my own Alcheringa. Look here. It's built to the standard Besa pattern of concrete hollow bricks, with a waiting room in the centre and a video player slung off the wall so people can watch health-promotion propaganda while they wait. Notice the four adults and one toddler. Young Faye and Young Edward and their older selves, Old Faye and Eddie Mayfield, all waiting for what the white doctor has to offer.

Blackfellas and whitefellas don't share a long history. The last of the Aborigines came in from the bush around 1987. Consistent interaction began in the early 1930s. Seventeen-year-old cameleer RM Williams, of Australian footwear fame, led missionaries into the Gibson Desert, built a water tank out of mud and moved on after a year. In walked the Aborigines, attracted by the constant supply of food and water. Missionaries began converting people, tried to stop their heathen ways and save the kids. Harsh climate and lack of food and water out bush in the late 1930s forced a lot of people to the mission. Some parents left their children with the men of the white spirit.

Interracial interaction only goes so far. Whitefellas aren't generally invited to certain ceremonies. Cultural traditions and beliefs – physical, spiritual and emotional survival information – are passed on progressively to boys as they age so they can take over. They have to know where the rock holes are and how to find water. Ceremonies are linked to the season, which means the availability of water and food. In November, the monsoons from the northwest of Western Australia spin down and across the Sandy and Gibson Deserts, bringing the rain that fills the soaks and rock holes. That way, the land can support more people, in groups of six to a dozen with one or two dominant males, three or four females, one or two older people and maybe two to four kids.

Here in this painting, Eddie Mayfield is talking to Old Faye, a woman from his skin group. The toddler of her younger self, Young Faye, is throwing plastic toys about the place, which all tolerate. Stocky Young Edward, who is Eddie 60 years ago, brandishes a crowbar at the door of the Besa brick building with one hand and spears a kangaroo with the other. That was the only way to do it in the old days, with a spear. A strict protocol determined how the 'roo was butchered, the bits into which he was cut and how that was distributed among the various members of the group. Quite often, the hunter got a fairly insubstantial share compared to other people in the group.

Notice Eddie's clothes. Very Western. Old Faye's wearing a bright-yellow sloppy T-shirt and long loose patterned shorts. Younger Faye's donned a red version of the same. Young Edward's stripped to the waist. I rarely saw him except for trauma injuries, perhaps a wound caused by a spear or a crowbar, like other young men in the community. Spearing can occur in the form of payback, weaving black justice into white man's rules.

Aborigines have easily accepted our food and clothing and the houses in which we live. They play videos, use PlayStations, smoke cigarettes and drive old Toyotas, Fords and Holdens. At the same time, they believe in spirits, or *mamus*. Sorcery.[7] It's one aspect of the strict protocols which guided traditional behaviour. Their traditional healers play a significant role in treating people. When someone presents with head, body or shoulder pain, I might suggest they go to the *nungkari*, the witch doctor. They might reply, 'I've been already and he took a sharp stick out of my body' or 'a stone out of my head.'

Eddie, Faye, Younger Faye and Young Edward are caught between a superstitious world view and our evidence-based one. Sometimes people present with fairly common problems, like gall- and kidney stones. I often wonder if the witch doctor can remove the stones.

Look at the next panel of the painting. Think I'll do a triptych, a revolving one that looks the same from all angles. We can't tell what the weather's doing in the first panel. Look at that sky! The purple lightning bolts and pummelling luminous raindrops are obvious, but can you tell that shaky lines are meant to be reverberating thunder?

Over here is Young Faye's consultation at the end of the day. Through that door off the waiting room is the consulting room. See the examining table spread with a clean white sheet, desk laden with such paraphernalia as steth and sphyg, and locked cabinets lining the walls. That's Faye in red and myself in a white shirt.

The rain eased and lightning split the sky.

---

7 They're not alone in this in the modern world. Look, for example, at a young Latina in Los Angeles, who claims that a *bruja* guided her gruesome murder of a snow-cone man in 2005. Available at: www.laweekly.com/2007-02-01/news/death-of-the-snow-cone-man (accessed 17 February 2012).

'What brings you in today?' I asked Young Faye.

'Got a goanna inside me,' came the reply. 'The witch doctor'll take that out.'

The goanna inside the young woman was sleight of hand, undoubtedly. People have shown me sticks that have been removed from them. Some were 10 or 12 centimetres long. You could see on the flat area where they'd been sharpened with a knife, so it was obviously a prepared object.

I leaned far forward to hear her over the waiting-room noise. It's challenging to act as a clinician in these communities, with different world views and high levels of hearing impairment and poverty causing childhood ear infections and perforated eardrums, in which a middle-ear infection bursts through. People often turn up the television quite loud. Dogs wander in or people yell during consultations, making it harder to listen to your patient's heart, or lungs or chest.

Being faced with such a presentation was a real paradox. This 19-year-old girl was smiling and happy to talk with me. She was a 'modern' Aboriginal teenager, but her belief system was worlds away from mine.

Her boy crawled, pulled himself up, walked tentatively and fell. He was fine and very healthy, thank God, because his mother was a social petrol sniffer who'd quit when she found out she was pregnant. A newish type of petrol being sold contains a different sort of hydrocarbon, so it doesn't have the same effect. A black market has developed, with sniffable petrol costing up to $50 a litre.

Thunder rumbled through the room. 'Some storm,' I said.

'A tree's burning,' Young Faye said.

'I'd like to have a look at it,' I said. We established its exact location on the outskirts of the community.

'It's wet,' she said, holding her child close and not looking at me directly.

'Can I give you a lift home in the Toyota?'

She nodded.

'Okay, but I'd like to drive over and see that tree first.'

'*Yuah*,' she said. Yes.

We buckled up in the troop carrier and I steered us across the spinifex to the flaming tree. A lightning strike was burning it at the base.

'Wonder why a bolt hit that particular tree,' I said. My neck was stiff so I stretched, side to side, eyes always forward. Faye appeared closer, farther, closer as my cervical vertebrae danced.

'A *mamu* was in that tree.'

'Why would a *mamu* be in that tree?'

'Aaahhh, somebody's been eating too much meat.'

I couldn't see the cause and effect, the relationship, but that was her explanation. Possibly there wasn't enough to go around so taking more than one's share was taboo.

I let it go at that. Patients can withdraw if you ask too many questions, if they perceive you as intrusive or too direct. Sometimes, I act a little obtuse, use an interpreter or go-between or talk in the third person.

Does *mamu* refer to one particular group of spirits? I don't know, but I do know a standard form of belief out here includes rainbow serpents that live in the desert in particular rock holes. Despite climatic extremes and changes, that story has been passed down from other groups elsewhere, in lusher parts of the country.

Green grass and soft earth b'long in another fella's Dreamtime. My colours are red, blue and yellow — your primary colours, doc — and black and white. Dirt, sky, the in-between . . . and men. Us and them. Me. You.

Next day during my lunch break, I walked down the street from the clinic to the arts centre. Old Faye'd had a dizzy spell. I fixed her up, but wanted to observe her for a little while, so I accepted a cup of tea and settled in to watch the day's proceedings. It was sale day. Art is one of the positive things happening in Aboriginal communities. People are painting and earning decent money, most of which stays with them.

One man gathered a lot of attention. He was the centre's externally funded coordinator, who provided paints and canvases and organised a place for artists to work. He also sold the paintings through recognised galleries in most of the capital cities. Individuals received most of the funds, minus a commission to fund the ongoing requirements of the art gallery and the coordinator. With him was the *punu* man, who comes from afar to buy bowls, carved snakes and figures decorated with burnt markings. He does it in an ethical way, to a standard formula: a bowl 300 millimetres long is worth this and a bowl 350 is worth that.

Old Faye got up shakily. '*Punu* man about my bowls,' she mumbled.

'I'm going back to the clinic, so I'll accompany you,' I said, taking her elbow.

Old Eddie Mayfield was talking to the buyer. Eddie was also a superb artist whose paintings fetched anything from $1000 to $6000. Eddie hasn't changed in any way whatsoever, even though he probably earns 30 or 40 thousand a year. He still wears daggy old clothes and drives an old Toyota. Probably a lot of the money he earns is disbursed through the extended family group because of traditional obligation–reciprocation. Does that foster dependency in some of the weaker males, or does it protect those unable to care for themselves, or perhaps a bit of both? Traditionally, a strict protocol dictated sharing of resources. I spear a kangaroo and have to butcher and distribute it a certain way. Unfortunately, pollution has crept in. Some younger people expect to receive money generated by artefacts and paintings that older people produce.

The *punu* man gave Faye $400 for her bowls. I steered her back to her seat and was heading out the door, back to the clinic, when three family members, a woman in her late teens and two young men – one of whom I recognised as Young Edward – bailed up my dizzy patient. They demanded that she give them some of the money she'd earned through her own efforts.

She complied. To me she said, without looking me in the eye, 'You go on without me, doc.'

To me, it's an unsuitable extension of a sharing tradition that was obviously functional in an extreme environment with minimal resources. Now it fostered inappropriate dependence in the younger ones. You don't need much imagination to see what this does to young men and women. It's another example of a hunter–gatherer society coming in from the cold (or the hot) within living memory that needs to restructure traditional behavioural protocols to meet modern demands. Artistic elders now may have more wealth to distribute than young men, upsetting the traditional way of things when protocol demands distribution upon demand.

Eddie turned away from the *punu* man and said, 'I'll be over later, doc.' He was fit except for a cough we were monitoring. Might do a lung-function test. He liked all the huffing and puffing, and it set a good example. When we first got the spirometer, many people presented with coughs.

With a last glance at Old Faye, I headed out the arts centre door and back to the clinic. Young Edward was arguing with another young man on the other side of the street. My heart sank. If he was on a petrol-sniffing bender, I'd be in trouble.

An English Christmas

Amaranth Fillet

If Uncle Zoltan hadn't plucked me up from the remotest locum on the planet and plunked me down in a medical conference in the Caribbean, I'd never have met Hubby Wayne. Who knows upon what shores the medical seas would have deposited me? Perhaps the land of research, tucked far away from other humans on a prison island or sleepy refugee lagoon. I may have tempted fate and opted for drug addicts, but I hope not: it was too raw and tempting until recently. Very recently. Desire occasionally spikes me, but I'm no longer willing to sacrifice the children. Or the husband. I don't delude myself. One minuscule lapse and all would be lost.

Out of a sea of faces, that goose-stepping procession of unpoetic suffering – mums and babes, the elderly, girls after the Pill, malingering young men angling for work certificates – out of all that, three faces loom large: Mrs Crumpacker and Reverend Eastley. And Mrs Eastley. All taught me something about being directionless and getting lost, my limitations and responsibilities as a locum and what life does to people. The consequences were momentous, both professionally and personally. I was there to hold the fort, not to fiddle with medications or attempt to change ingrained behaviour.

One Christmas shortly after we were married, Wayne and I were doing a locum in London. Enter Mrs Crumpacker, creaking and groaning as she blew in with the bad weather. The old darling attended our practice from a nearby one. In the UK, that was a big thing. I heard her haranguing other patients in the waiting room as I went to get my next patient.

'. . . so far from the bus and such a long footpath, dear. I'm not well, I tell you, not at all well. I don't know how much longer I can wait.'

I called out, 'Mrs Crumpacker?'

The old lady eyeballed me and grunted reproachfully, 'It will take me time to get up, doctor. I've waited so long, me bones have gone stiff.'

'Take your time.'

'I intend to.' She was short and angular with hair drawn tightly back, accentuating her stony expression.

Bringing up the rear on the long march to the consulting room provided enough time to question my vision of the future. I yearned for the darker side of life with patients who fell through the cracks, like Olyce Parp, a reluctant thief who, before he robbed them, prayed for forgiveness to the Japanese couple that always left out best-quality green tea for their irregular visitor.

I summoned all my resources for Tank of Crone crunching inexorably ahead of me. After some time, she colonised the consulting room. If you discounted the obvious, that she was a whingeing old tyrant, she actually did describe symptoms of polymyalgia.

'We'll just take some blood, Mrs Crumpacker, and have you fixed up for Christmas.'

'I don't think I'll live, doctor, not with this pain.' Her tightly pulled hair accentuated a sloping forehead.

'Well, ring up and we'll always fit you in.'

'That's another thing, doctor. Your staff.' Her hard face became even stonier, her lips tightly compressed.

I tuned out.

'. . . rude on the phone, the way they give directions . . . wonder I didn't end up in Scotland, especially that young redhead, she's a bad 'un. I can tell.'

I nodded. Because she complained so much, I held off putting her on prednisolone until I was sure of my diagnosis. 'We'll wait for your results before we start you on tablets.'

I heard from the lab 3 days later, on Christmas Eve. Suspicions confirmed. I pitied her regular GP, poor bastard. I'd ferret her out and bestow her prescription and a bottle of tablets; otherwise, she'd have to wait until after Christmas, and they worked so fast.

I set off, through densely populated southeast England and its obscure little lanes. Roads changed their names from Something Close to Something Lane. Our road sported three number twos; our house exhibited no number but was called Montague Cottage.

For one so rudderless, I've been proficient at picking my way through back lanes and paddocks searching for poorly lit and badly marked houses. You lose so much time and possibly a life searching for a house with no identification. It was worse in England. No blankets over hedges led me to Mrs Crumpacker. With some difficulty, I found the road leading to the lane to the byway to her house. A bland young man answered my knock.

'I'm Dr Fillet. Is Mrs Crumpacker in?'

'Who?'

'Mrs . . .' I consulted the prescription, 'Agnes Crumpacker.'

'No one here by that name,' said the young man in the usual stilted English manner. They are inordinately polite because you're a doctor and class consciousness is ground into them from an early age.

'Oh. She came to the surgery the day before yesterday and gave this address.'

'I'll get Mum. Please come in.'

'Thanks, mate.'

I waited in the cold dark hallway until a middle-aged lady appeared.

'My son didn't know,' apologised that stout woman. 'His sister, my daughter, got married in October. Her husband's grandmother came with them.'

'Here's a prescription for Mrs Crumpacker, and some tablets to keep her going until it's filled.'

'This way, please, doctor.'

We started off to the parlour. Halfway down the dark passageway, the lady of the house turned back to me and said hopefully, 'Have you come to take her to hospital?'

'No, to calm her down so she doesn't suffer over Christmas.'

A young woman and an attentive young man, obviously the newlyweds, wheeled in the old lady.

'Hello, Mrs Crumpacker, how . . .'

'I've still got that pain in me shoulder, doctor,' Mrs Crumpacker complained, without so much as a hello.

'I've brought you some tablets that should fix you right up.'

Mrs Crumpacker's paw swiped at them. She didn't say a word. The young man leaned forward and guided the plastic bottle into her hand. He pocketed the prescription. Nobody said anything, nor offered me a cup of tea, nor thanked me for coming. They nodded politely, in that English way they use before they shoot the neighbours.

'Well, I'll be off,' I said, finally. 'Happy Christmas.'

I hurried down the footpath, face towards a damp London winter, judging ungenerously.

'Wait, doctor!' The bride bustled after me with some Australian wine. 'My husband and I wanted you to have this.' She handed me the bottle.

It must have finally dawned on her that I'd gone incredibly out of my way and done something considerate for this old woman, for whom I reckon the milk of human kindness had dried up 50 years earlier.

'Happy Christmas,' said the newly married girl, 'and thank you.'

Mrs Crumpacker was probably perfectly ordinary in her youth. To this day, I think of her if I find myself grousing too much.

Our second locum in England provided another cautionary tale of limitations and consequences. Two weeks in a sleepy village should nicely round off our medical experience of the mother country. Wayne and I shot down to Kent the day after I delivered Mrs Crumpacker's prescription and tablets. We'd heard of all sorts of strange people living 20 miles from London, in that enclave where well-to-do Londoners kept their mistresses in the 1930s and 1940s. Lloyd George supposedly hid his girlfriends down there. One rumour ensconced Ethel Leneuve, beloved of the wife-murdering dentist Crippin, in a modest little cottage on the high street. The men had long since died, but some of the mistresses were still alive – stranded elderly ladies, the remains of romance. The village straddled a valley. When it snowed – up to 13 inches deep – our principal closed the surgery and visited patients in their homes.

I couldn't wait to nibble the edges of conventionality through to the core. I can control the inclination now, at least externally, but the need remains. Rodently gnaws into the Normandy Camembert of respectability were all I could trust myself with, all I had left to propitiate my demons. My new husband and new life – not to mention my work – unfolded before me along a ribbony highway. It took all my energy to drive that road and not crash.

Our employer, the village doctor, advised introducing ourselves to the local Anglican priest, so off we set one frigid mid-morning to Reverend Eastley on his small farm at the edge of the village. A matronly woman answered our ring and led us into the parlour. Her frizzy hair and general pallor supported her air of partial recovery from a debilitating illness that left her bruised and cheated by life. 'The vicar will be right with you, doctors,' she said, leading us into a tiny sitting room-cum-library. 'He's finishing up some correspondence.'

I browsed the bookcases peppering the walls. Ah, here was an omnivorous owner who examined his theology from many angles. Political biographies and thinkers predominated. Photographs perched in front of the books, of children advancing through life, crawling, toddling, running in school sports and finally immobile at the altar. Proud Mum threaded through them.

The vicar's wife settled us on the settee with Christmas cake, weak tea and assurances that her husband wouldn't be long. I was forcing my weather-numbed fingers round the delicate handle of a transparent china cup when in fluttered a personage as grey and white as the pigeons we heard cooing out the back. He sat down across from us, a picture of neatness. Trouser creases knife-blade crisp. Nary a shirt wrinkle anywhere. The quality of his apparel was astonishing for a man of the cloth.

I liked him immediately. How personal religion was in British villages. If I lived there, I'd become a practicing Christian of his denomination just to be in his orbit.

'So glad to meet you, dear I mean doctor,' he said to me. He'd a cheerful expression and eyes that missed nothing, accustomed to assessing but not judging. 'I've always wanted to chat with someone intelligent from your country. Avian matters fascinate me.'

'I haven't much time for birdwatching,' I replied.

Wayne clucked beside me. 'Ask her about rock and roll.' I was grateful for his body warmth in the chilly parlour. 'Anything at all.'

'One would think those scarlet-and-turquoise parrots are quite hip,' he observed. 'And those monotremes and marsupials. At one time, we almost emigrated.'

'But we'd the children to think of.' Mrs Eastley finished his sentence in the way of long-married couples.

'And Margaret here didn't want to leave her family.'

A look flashed across her face that spoke of a victory hard won for which she still paid. Our principal had told us about the full plate of the vicar's wife, which made her a compulsive bargain hunter obsessed with being short-changed. My limitations as a locum chafed. Our employer was telling me only enough to keep my finger in the dyke. Apparently, Mrs Eastley weighed her groceries as soon as she got home from the market and shopped tirelessly to find the best price on the smallest goods. She was happy to travel some distance for a bargain – it was exercise – and didn't bother about time being money.

The vicar leaned over and patted my hand. 'You'll be fine, dear.'

I'd no doubts until he spoke, but now I wondered.

I was on call a few nights later when the phone rang around eleven. My hand shot out reflexively from Wayne Warmth under the blankets to claw the bedside table before clamping on the receiver.

'It's Mrs Eastley, doctor. Sorry to disturb you, but my husband is acting strangely. Can you come out to the farm?'

I jumped into the principal's Land Rover, which he insisted we use despite protestations of our Volkswagen's magical powers. I mourned its sound system as I stoked up the heater, slotted in an old tape of 'Good Golly Miss Molly' – if that didn't wake me up, nothing would – and sallied forth into the night. I blasted the heater on full. Winters in that part of southeast England were hideous. Cold, snow and wind created a whole worse than the sum of its parts.

The distressed spouse met me at the front door in her bathrobe, which she clenched tight at the throat. 'He's becoming like his father. First he stops sleeping, then he won't sit still.'

Following the manic vicar from room to room soon warmed me up. I gripped my black bag all the while. He was unbelievably scruffy. Was it only 3 days since we met? Creased trousers, open-necked shirt missing a button. Day-old stubble. Hair standing up on his scalp. He was fairly coherent despite talking nineteen to the dozen, as people can be in the manic phase of bipolar illness.

'I'm going to send a letter to the prime minister and include a mousetrap,' he said in the kitchen. 'What he's doing overseas is wrong' . . . striding into the passageway . . . 'no, it's unconscionable' . . . flinging open the door of the closet-sized study . . . '"All that is necessary for the triumph of evil is that good men do nothing." Edmund Burke. I can't keep quiet any longer' . . . taking the stairs two at a time . . . 'I've got a responsibility to my flock.'

I sympathised with his politics and moral dilemma and momentarily considered adding my name to his letter but decided that would be unwise. 'As do I, vicar. I'm going to give you something to calm you down.'

His wife and I popped the distressed citizen into bed, and I left.

It seemed that I'd just fallen asleep when the phone jangled. The bedside clock assured me that several hours had snuck away.

'Doctor,' whispered the vicar's wife, 'he's vanished!'

The short drive back to the farm was bitterly cold.

'The kitchen window's open,' Mrs Eastley said, shivering, as soon as I arrived.

'I'll have a look,' I said.

'No, wait until that young constable arrives. My husband can be, well . . .' She clutched her bathrobe round her middle and phoned the police. She put down the receiver and explained, 'He was the brilliant one in the family, but was unable to defy his father. He never wanted to be a vicar. He feels as if his life is wasted.'

'That must be hard for you.'

Her expression told me I didn't know the half of it.

The constable arrived remarkably quickly given the weather conditions. The three of us formed a knot in the garden out the back. 'You go inside, Mother, the doc 'n I'll find him.' She complied gratefully. The hunt was on. What Mr Eastley called his farm was a few chooks and a shed constructed of corrugated iron and barbed wire. We followed the sound of loud cooing and found him crouching in a coop, fondling a pigeon. Under his dressing gown, the vicar wore street clothes in unspeakable disarray. 'I'm verifying something for my letter to the prime minister, doctor, and I think best like this,' he said.

Little Richard invaded me, singing 'I got the heeby jeebies and I can't get well.' 'You may have caught a chill out here in this weather. It's best if we take you in for observation.'

'But the police . . .'

'Your wife rang them because she was concerned. I'll meet you at the hospital and we'll start you on some tablets that will do you the world of good.'

The vicar was perfectly polite. 'That's very kind of you, but I prefer my mind to be clear.'

I knew what he meant. I hated to flatten his highs and understood his need to spice up his life. The usual ways – sex, drugs and rock and roll – were closed to an honourable man in his circumstances.

Perhaps I'd have acted differently if I'd been his permanent GP and we hadn't his wife to consider. I couldn't, tempting as it was. I'd certain responsibilities as a locum. We eventually got him into the police car, the liveliness sliding from his eyes. The manifestations of his approaching low would fall upon his wife's shoulders. Again. I kept him in hospital to give her a preparatory rest.

I made the time during our village rounds to pop out and check that her needs didn't drown in the minutiae of her husband's illness. 'How are you holding up?' I asked one morning over weak tea and Christmas cake at the kitchen table. Relentless snow swirled outside the window above the sink, flakes clinging to bare black branches. The extreme-white quality of light turned my hostess as pale as the milk in the jug before us.

'Thank you for keeping him in hospital, doctor,' she said, nibbling a crumb or two. 'Gives me a chance to rest – not that I don't miss him, of course.'

'Of course.'

'You've no idea how bad he can get.' A defeated look pulled her eyes at the corners.

'Have you spoken to Dr __?' I named our principal.

'Men don't always understand, in my experience.' She put her hand on mine. 'Do you have to leave our village, dear?'

For once, Little Richard was silent. I wanted to stay forever. 'I've my husband to consider,' I said, copping out with the first trickle in a convenient torrent of spouse blaming.

She nodded. Sadly. She knew. I felt diminished.

'I'll see if Wayne agrees to our doing another locum here next Christmas.' How to Avoid the Neurotic Jollity of Family Celebrations, Plan A.

'Do your best, dear. I'll manage.' Her generosity in extreme adversity made my eyes tear. Not for the last time, a patient put me to shame.

Mr Eastley was still in hospital when we left.

Our principal said that the vicar's wife had a heart of gold. He always came away with a dozen eggs, and I was no eggs-ception, despite the cold. Mrs Eastley died before I could return. I kept meaning to, for years. I've never forgiven Wayne for that.

It comes by air ▄▄▄▄

Wayne Cooperville

'Some words descend unbidden when I recall meeting my wife by the foghorn: gush, rush, cascade, spurt, jet, fume, churn, ferment, seethe, boil and flammable,' Wayne said. We were in his shed out the back. 'Remember these?' he asked, hammering the wooden shutters from the decayed seaside bar. 'Married medical life has me in its velvet grip. Mirages from night-time seas no longer come a-calling. Nor do I feel shame for letting down my literary heroes with besotted responses to women. My passion for cryptozoology finds me at the end of a periscope rather than on deck. I've never been happier.'

All sorts of health hazards ripple the surface of rural life in the twenty-first century, such as the ever-present unemployment, underemployment and self-employment, with their clusters of problems like boredom and low self-esteem. These lead to scorching abuse directed inward, in the form of alcoholism and suicide, and aimed outward in a deluge of spouse beating. Darren Blinty's father barely harnessed a fiery temper that both imploded and exploded.

After our locum in England, we fell by chance into a city practice, near the one in which Amaranth's Uncle Zoltan worked when he took her on a home visit to Olyce Parp, the thief she particularly liked. After 5 years or so, our practice took over a rural run about 45 minutes' drive away, from a GP who had simply closed up shop and returned to Ireland to nurse his dying mother. Amaranth and I jumped at the chance to divvy up the remote duties. Our colleagues were thrilled. So were we, except for one thing: my wife wanted to work for a month or two in Sussex to be with Mrs Eastley, the vicar's wife.

So began our association with the Blintys. The only jobs available in the country are often unskilled and badly paid. That was nothing new. The sense of life passing one by isn't as pronounced now, with satellite television and the Internet. However, those modern wonders spawn their own brand of bedevilment as people compare their lot with what's on the screen. Something else hasn't changed: lower incomes and lack of access to services. A yoga teacher once commented that his city students had more flexibility and his country ones more strength. Darren Blinty was able to drag himself to work despite being drenched with toxic chemicals by an aerial sprayer, which he always claimed resulted in significant neurological impairment. Here was a taboo subject: exposure to farm chemicals.

Darren Blinty acceded to his father's wishes and joined him in the family business. Mrs Blinty always looked on the bright side and was reassured that her son wasn't working in the mines. Darren had the rotten luck to be sprayed twice by aerial crop dusters. He called me the day after the second drenching.

'I don't trust myself to drive, doc, but I'm prob'ly okay.'

'I'm coming that way later. You keep warm by the fire. I'll be there as soon as I can.' Examinations were easier to do in the surgery, but I wanted to spare the poor man the trouble. He'd been through enough.

When it started 2 years ago, Darren Blinty was a 33-year-old fencing contractor working next to a Forestry Department tree plantation. 'One day, I heard a rumble, a crop duster overhead. I didn't think anything of it. In fact, I waved, and the pilot flashed his lights back.'

Darren lived alone in a little weatherboard cottage on the edge of one of those tiny towns which populate our state. His house belonged to the landscape in a way that signalled deep connection with centuries past. I wound my way round the shrubs to the front door. No rose bushes here: Darren's late mother gave up *that* battle years before her death, finally yielding to the inevitability of possums. A struggle with the forces of nature, cleanly fought, didn't bother her, unlike chemical spraying and logging and the unfair advantages they gave humans. Last time I saw her, she pronounced herself weary of imprisoning the rose bushes behind stakes and wire. She'd grown to admire her enemy. I glanced at the bedroom on the right. The window coverings drooped, berating me: How could I let this awful thing happen?

'Leave your boots on, doc.' Darren was interrupted by the jerking of his arm in a backward lash from the elbow, flicking away a giant insect. 'Now that Mum's gone, I can do anything I want.' Some victories are pyrrhic.

I followed a body clothed in a blue, black and white plaid flannel shirt and olive-green work pants into the lounge room.

'Ever considered marrying, Darren? I can recommend it.' I couldn't bring myself to say that he might need care in the not-too-distant future.

'Once I pondered it, but I like being able to eat dinner when I want and not be ragged at about table manners.'

'I can understand that, Darren, but it's a high price to pay for small pleasures.'

'They're the best kind,' he said. A beatific smile spread over his face. 'Noticed you looking at the curtains. Can't keep up with 'em since Mum died.'

Darren's father settled with the mining company, to which he had devoted his working life, after a loader pinned him against the rock face underground. He purchased this 3-acre block and started up as a fencing contractor. His son took over the business 8 years ago.

'Sit here, doc.' Darren dislodged a well-worn copy of Giovanni Caselli's *The Roman Empire and the Dark Ages* and indicated a weary sofa near the wood fire. Raggedly ripped strips of paper marked many of the pages. Home visits were a continual revelation. He noticed my surprise.

'I like learning about daily life in the old days, especially the tools they used,' he said, sitting next to me. 'It all started when Mum read me the story when I was this high' – he pointed at his knees – 'of that little blind boy and his dog in Pompeii when Vesuvius erupted.'

Mrs Blinty was a schoolteacher known for her love of reading and collection of tea towels. I wondered what had happened to them and made a mental note to enquire another time. I couldn't imagine he'd any use for them. Local gossip spied no women on his horizon, but you never knew.

'Imagine watching your uncle cark it. That's what happened, you know, sort of, when Vesuvius erupted. First Uncle Pliny wanted to go over and investigate because he was a scientist, but then he got a call of distress from a lady friend so he hurried to rescue her. His nephew waited across the bay, but the older man was either overcome by gases or suffered a heart attack. He never returned.'

Darren knew what it was like to wait in vain for a male relative. His father shot himself with a .22 behind the shed.

'How are you feeling, Darren?'

'Got me, didn't they?'

He meant the tree plantation on state government land, a monoculture experiment that environmentalists claimed courted disaster. They set baits using 1080 to annihilate possums and other animals that ate the seedlings. The crop duster sprayed alpha-cypermethrin, which killed beetles on eucalyptus leaves.

'You know me, doc. Fit as a flea before all this started.' And that was the truth. 'I started to feel dizzy in the beginning, the first time I was sprayed.'

'And the little tics?'

'Wasn't long before they came, doc. You might remember as you made me go to that torture doctor in the city.'

I'd sent Darren to a neurologist, who found nothing and requested toxicology tests. We sent interstate for that. Our remoteness is a double-edged sword when it comes to sophisticated laboratory tests or anything out of the ordinary.

Darren got caught in the middle of the volcanic debate about the effects of aerial spraying on our water catchments that erupted between powerful business forces and everybody else with any sanity. The former included those venal or ignorant enough to be bought off or seduced by the hem of power, including some of our government officials and battlers like Darren Blinty – BS, before spraying.

'I always thought the Greenies were mad, doc. Now I wonder. It took all my strength to get myself well enough so's I could work part-time.' No histrionics, only a countryman determined to do his job.

'If all my patients were as healthy as you, I'd be out of business.'

Here it was, the twitching human face of disaster.

'Tell me about the last time you were sprayed.'

He put another log on the fire, settled in and started to talk. 'I was out the Helston place. They're new round here. They were paying top dollar. I needed the money.'

I knew the family. Mrs Pru H brought in the children regularly and demanded a suburban style of practice. Olivia and Jack contracted the usual childhood ailments. Their mother displayed the superior air of those who considered themselves as adventurous as Mawson and Hillary for moving from town to country. They planned to continue growing their predecessor's chestnut trees injected with truffle mould. On their backblocks, they were running sheep for lavender ice cream, a new gourmet goodie. If they stayed long enough, their city patina would erode. Meanwhile, their outrage at being duped into envisioning themselves as pioneers in a pristine wilderness might translate into activism. We needed people on our side with financial interests in cleaning up our environment and no social ties pulling the other way.

'Let me look at your pupils.' I drew in close. 'Now screw up your eyes.'

He complied. 'It's getting worse, doc,' he said, glancing at the fire as a log crackled.

'Let's see what we can do. Turn your head from side to side.'

'Must have been like being gassed in the first war. I heard that plane comin'.'

One side.

'There was nowhere to run. I sometimes wake up in the night with that sound in me head and knowin' what's coming.'

The other.

'And the awful feelin' that comes in nightmares, the helplessness.'

Another jerk interrupted his speech.

When he settled down, he said, 'By the way, doc, think your wife'd like Mum's tea towels?'

Visions of a domesticated Amaranth contentedly drying dishes raised a smile. 'I'm not sure she's the right person to appreciate that sort of gift. Now shrug your shoulders. Well done. Why not donate them to the church raffle?'

'Did you know, doc, that in the first stage, dust, ashes, cinders and rocks spewed out from Vesuvius for many miles around? I think of that as the warning. It happened well before the hot steam and boiling mud came flowing. It only took 4 minutes for the boiling mud from Vesuvius to travel 7 kilometres to the nearest town.'

I got out the reflex hammer. 'Don't send me back to the torture man, doctor.'

'I won't. One little test and that'll be it.'

'What am I gonna do? I can't sit around all day reading about burning mountains.'

'Did the Forestry respond to your letter?'

'Yeah, and they basically said it wasn't their fault.'

'I wish I had an answer for you, Darren. We'll have to wait and see.'

'This is my life we're talking about! Don't they care?'

'Market forces,' I began, and stopped. This wasn't the time to discuss chemical and environmental devastation.

His anger ebbed, and he sagged into the sofa. 'I know how Dad felt at the end.'

A farmer's demons and Hughie's angels

Malcolm Phillips

'Thank you for coming, ladies and gentlemen of the press. I'm pleased to announce, as the newly appointed president of our esteemed state medical association, that I have successfully lobbied the federal government for funds to increase mental health care. Among other things, we will now be remunerated adequately for extremely long home visits.'

Some things never change, like distressed wives and out-of-control husbands. Madness stared me in the face in both country and town. Alcohol and isolation exacerbated my farmer's condition and quite possibly my urban madman's. Both wives stood by their men through life's downward spirals. I learned one lesson early on as a young general practitioner: if there's trouble, you don't go looking for it. It will find you soon enough.

New Zealand. Dead of winter. Late July. Long ago. Late at night. Raining like mad. I got a call to an old farmhouse quite a distance from my village, in the district of another young doctor. The man of the house had gone mad – stark, raving bonkers.

'Can you help me out on this one?' my colleague pleaded. He'd rung me straight away, from a neighbouring practice. He was paying back the government for his medical education with the required 2 years of servitude in a rural area. Doctors hated it. He was no different. They'd do their 2 years and be off. Compulsion in rural practice is just not on. I'd left England and was on my way to Australia, with a stopover in the Land of the Long White Cloud because a friend needed me.

In that weather, it took me an hour to drive the 30 miles into the bush, to a place with a Maori name. I finally arrived at the farmhouse in the driving rain. There was nothing between the Antarctic and me. Foveaux Strait off the South Island is one of the four stormiest straits in the Southern Hemisphere. The wind howls in from Antarctica, as on that night.

I walked round to the back door, which was open.

'Hello,' I called into the house. No response.

I looked at my watch. Just gone nine. Maybe the woman of the house was putting the little ones to bed.

'It's the doctor,' I called, louder. Still no response. I pushed through the door into the kitchen. A fire roared. Comfortable chairs were nearby. Not a soul in sight. In the distance, I heard yells and shouts, dogs barking and other noise of the chase. Bugger it. Why should I join the search for a madman on a night like this? A few years earlier, I'd have done so and got soaked to the skin. I'd be no use to my patients if I caught a raging cold.

I considered myself a moderately experienced GP with eyes on a city practice, so I stoked up the fire, sat down in the most comfortable chair and waited. The immaculate room with its ineffable smells set me to marvelling at the cleanliness of New Zealand farmers' wives. As in so many others, a massive wooden table dominated the room, 2 metres long by 1.5 metres wide, scrubbed to perfection. The dishes were all beautifully racked.

This sent me into a spasm of silent appreciation for wives in general and my own in particular. I'm constantly amazed at what they put up with. In all my years in medicine, I have encountered quite a lot of cases in which women stay with men through all adversities – drinking, gambling and much, much worse – but little of the other way round. Abusive partners are almost always male.

If a GP is extremely lucky, he ends up with a first-rate spouse. I'd go so far as to identify that as one of the most important ingredients, if not *the* most important, of a successful medical career. She can feed the flames or extinguish them. What constitutes good? It's relative, as moral imperatives so often are. She does not have a demanding profession, but places the needs of her husband first and foremost, always ahead of her own. She must be happy with her own company, not require her spouse's physical presence, and sometimes not his emotional one. She must think of them as a team. She must often put up with lack of respect from the world at large, which perceives her as privileged, idle and materialistic. In countries with socialised medicine, she must manage on a limited household budget, and do so with a smile because no one wants to hear a doctor's wife complaining. What decided me to marry my dear wife was reading in her diary before we married – accidentally, of course – how she accounted for every ha'penny spent. That's my girl.

Such ruminations occupied my mind for three quarters of an hour, when frenzied sounds in the distance intruded into the absolute quiet of the kitchen. The posse cornered the farmer. I heard each nuance of the hunt as canine and human sounds approached. Looking back, it was highly amusing.

The wife materialised first, absolutely saturated. Her mad husband soon appeared, restrained by his two sons, the doctor and a farmhand. Husband and wife looked like brother and sister, big-boned, fair and florid and pulsing with physical health. The difference was in the eyebrows. His were white-blonde and bushy, meeting in the middle. Hers were honey-coloured and pencil-thin, arching well into her forehead with a rather surprised look. Or was it disdain when she looked at me?

They had pursued the farmer until he fell into a ditch full of water. They hauled him back, drenched and dripping weeds like a tree with epiphytes, like Spanish moss in the oaks of the American Deep South. All were filthy and soaked to the skin. Rain pounded on the corrugated iron roof.

'Why didn't you join us?' demanded my aggrieved colleague.

'No need. You caught him and brought him back.'

'You weren't called on to sit in front of a fire.'

'Enough bods were after him, and you got him in the ditch anyway,' I said, refusing to allow his irritability to dispel the warmth. 'You want me to run around like a dog. As Hercule Poirot told Captain Hastings in *The ABC Murders*, my force is in my brains, not my feet.'

The farmer's wife faded into the background, perhaps to change out of her wet clothes, leaving a gaggle of men in the kitchen. We two doctors did not hesitate to certify the violent, screaming farmer. The problem was to subdue him. In those days, you used phenobarb. I injected, which cooled him off considerably. The problem was carting him to the nearest mental hospital, which was 200 miles away. His sons bundled him into a car and drove with my colleague to the nearest town, where they swapped over and an ambulance took him off.

I was gone 4 hours, from eight to after midnight, and returned home nice and dry to my waiting wife.

I was fortunate to have finished my medical training in less pressurised times. Nowadays, extraneous values and politics force students to choose a specialty at least as early as halfway through medical school. I don't approve of this Balkanisation of the health professions. It's become very difficult for members of these proliferating and centrifugal specialties to communicate with their colleagues in other fields, not to mention their patients, and for patients to navigate a confident pathway among this bewildering array of specialised branches of practice, each with its unique and dazzling high-tech impedimenta. I pity the poor medical graduate who, having embarked upon a particular specialist track, wants to change to another specialty, like many of my contemporaries. That's a lesson from evolution: a species that specialises in order to cope with a particular environment is endangered when that environment changes.

We used to say that a quarter of the knowledge we acquired in medical school would be obsolete or proved wrong within 10 years. Now the numbers have changed, and half of all medical knowledge has to be reappraised, revised or discarded, and in 5 years.

Shortly after I'd emigrated here and become a junior partner in a city practice, I inherited a husband and wife who resembled one another, in mannerisms more than build.

Hughie Weed's wife rang in a panic just after lunch one day. My senior partner had the call put through to me.

'It's his angels, doctor,' Mrs Weed explained.

Usually, daytime house calls were quite routine and straightforward. As the newest doctor, I was lowest in the pecking order, so naturally it was I who took that call. Ah, a first-class opportunity to prove my worth.

I rushed out, found the house and knocked smartly. While I was waiting, I admired a sailing ship etched into the front door's central glass panel.

The lady of the house finally peeked out. 'Oooh, you're the doctor. I'm Mrs Weed.'

'What seems to be the problem?' I asked.

Two vertical, deeply ingrained worry lines carved the face of the woman, dead centre between the eyes, as if someone had fired potshots at her frontal lobe.

'Oooh, good, doctor, I'm so glad you're here. Come in,' she said, gesturing me inside.

With that, she disappeared, like the farmer's wife in New Zealand. A door latched gently in the back of the house, loosening the aroma of heating soup. I was marooned in the passageway, which was not nearly as clean and inviting as the mad farmer's kitchen. The hallway was notable for its absence of furniture. No telephone table, umbrella tree, coat pegs, hatstand; indeed, no moveable ornament that could be thrown at or hide angels. Red and blue side windows dominated the front door. A galleon etched in glass sailed across the top. Old crimson carpet fraying at the edges and threadbare in the middle snaked down the centre of the floor, leaving 3 inches of scuffed wood on either side. A glass lotus shade shielded the single light bulb overhead.

I heard sounds in one of the rooms. I entered, and pulled the covers back to reveal a man lying fully clothed in his cap and boots. Freckles bespattered his cheek ridge like a happy starfield. His desiccated build and distressed expression mirrored his wife's. He possessed the same furrowed brow with two mournfully etched vertical wrinkles. I've seen such unlikely occurrences more than once. The couple appeared to be in late middle age, but it can be difficult to tell sometimes with those who have suffered more than their share.

'Good day,' said I, being a polite person. 'You must be Mr Weed.'

Hughie sat up and looked me in the eye, brows knitting. 'Who are you?'

'I'm the doctor,' I answered crisply.

'You've come for the angels.' Hughie leapt out of bed and took me firmly by the elbow. 'This way,' he said. 'On the tops of picture frames.'

There I was, in my best suit, clutching my doctor's bag and stethoscope and being ushered out of a bedroom to seek celestial beings.

I accompanied Hughie into the lounge, with a sofa and chair and wall-to-wall prints at waist height. They were all of a painting, with only an inch between them.

'Nicolas Poussin,' he said, '*Landscape with a Calm*.'

'Ah, seventeenth-century French classical landscape painting,' I said, for something to say.

My host approached the first picture and said, 'What colour's that one?'

I hesitated.

'Can't you see them?' he demanded.

'No. Where are they?'

'Just up there.' He pointed to the top of the frame.

I hesitated.

'What colour are they?' he repeated belligerently.

'I'm not sure,' I said.

'I want to know between red and black,' Hughie prompted.

'Red,' I responded. Black angels were probably unwelcome.

'Red angels,' he said, mollified. 'Right.' He pulled me by the elbow to the next picture. We circled the room, from picture to picture, assigning colours to invisible angels. Meanwhile, patients were piling up back at the surgery.

Suddenly, his hands tightened on me. 'What's wrong, Mr Weed?'

'That's not the right colour, doc. You're not seeing my cherubs correctly.' He picked me up by the scruff of the neck and the seat of the pants and threw me out of the house. To this day, I don't know how he accomplished it, given the disparity in our heights. Here I was, rapidly sailing towards the glass galleon on the front door and bracing myself to go straight through it.

Considerately, Hughie set me down outside before that could happen.

What to do now?

I ran next door and begged to use their telephone, claiming a medical emergency. I rang the surgery and spoke to my senior partner, who advised, 'Call the police.'

The neighbour gave me directions to the police station, which fortunately wasn't too far away. Alacrity of police access is one big difference between bush and city life. A massive sergeant was sitting at the desk.

I explained the circumstances. 'The man is obviously deranged,' I said. 'He needs to go to hospital.'

'Sure, doc,' the sergeant said, rising. 'No problem. I'll come along.'

'Wait! I don't think you're allowed to arrest somebody and cart him off just like that.'

''e's been rude to you, 'asn't 'e, doc?'

'Well, not exactly rude. He's mentally ill.'

'I'd better get the inspector.'

He fetched that personage, who agreed there was a Mental Health Act.

To commit someone in those days, you went before a magistrate and swore a warrant for arrest. We intervened in the middle of a special hearing and arranged to apprehend Hughie Weed.

'The patient is probably plain, ordinary mad,' I told the magistrate. 'It's a rarish condition, but it does occur.'

I was starting to doubt the whole thing. If you stand up and say you've been looking at red and black angels on the tops of picture frames in a magistrate's court, he'll probably think that it is you who should be hospitalised, especially if you add that all the paintings are the same and placed at waist height.

We eventually obtained the warrant. Our little procession – the sergeant, the inspector and myself – set off to Hughie Weed's house.

We knocked.

'Good day, gentlemen,' said Hughie Weed in his sanest voice. 'What can I do for you?'

The inspector looked at me.

'I'm sorry, Mr Weed,' I said, 'but we have a warrant for you to go to hospital.'

'Why?' he asked, genuinely puzzled.

'You were acting very strangely before,' I answered weakly.

'But I've never seen you before.'

'Ah,' said the inspector.

Silence.

'Look, you've got a warrant, you've gone to considerable trouble, and in my opinion, this man is mad,' I said to the inspector. 'I think you have to act on this opinion and sort it out at the hospital.'

'All right,' the inspector agreed reluctantly.

In a deep gruff voice, the sergeant, who was well over 6 feet tall, said to the shrunken patient, 'Will you come with me.' He phrased it as a question, but issued it as a command.

'Yes, certainly,' Hughie replied, completely compliant.

So they all trooped off.

This house call consumed 3 hours. I was exhausted when I got back to the surgery. Now I faced explanations to my colleagues and afternoon surgery.

Around 5:00, the psychiatric registrar rang me up. 'Mr Hugh R Weed is in here, and he's perfectly normal. He's agreed to go to bed for observation overnight.' Pause. I knew what was coming. 'You're sure of your diagnosis?'

'Well, in my opinion, he's mad,' I said.

The psychiatric registrar heaved a big doubting sigh. 'All right.'

The next morning, I rang up the hospital in fear and trembling. To my great joy, I ascertained that Hughie Weed had assaulted the nurses through the night on the grounds that they refused to look after the angels properly. He'd been smartly removed to the local mental hospital.

My honour was satisfied. I never saw Hughie Weed again. He came at his isolation from a different angle than the New Zealand farmer, but the end result was the same: they were both carted off and locked away, leaving their steadfast wives to pick up the pieces.

Boorish geese and ▬▬▬
car horns

Dexter Veriform

'Hello doctor, you're late,' Dexter Veriform said, squirming in his hospital bed. 'I need more of your magic bullets for the pain. As with home visits, there's a certain expectation on both sides that the doctor will arrive expeditiously. Being unreasonably late, in addition to the obvious consequences, can show disrespect or lack of caring. Being too early catches people unawares. Some doctors may prefer this, but I like to give my patients the time they need to secure their psychic armour, patients like Nicky Doulton-Brown's Mrs Dymphna O'Reilly, who insisted on the doctor visiting at 8 a.m. each Tuesday. It gave form to her week and a sense of control in an increasingly powerless existence. Once I received a gift from a grateful family member after a callout to which I was unconscionably late, through no fault of my own.'

I've never held anything back. Perhaps I shouldn't have shown so much emotion with my patients, like the day I prayed to the ringing telephone not to interfere with lunch, just this once. I'd spent the morning at an outpost surgery in Mile High, 13 miles from my practice at Banded Plover in New Zealand, after Olive and I had left the west coast of Scotland. I didn't particularly like going to these outpost surgeries. By the time I finished the clinic and the inevitable house calls and raced home for a bite of lunch, the waiting room would be full and the patients fidgeting. I was behind before I started. Invariably, a farm accident required accurate stitching as soon as I called in the first patient.

Summer settled upon us that early December day. I ushered out my last patient after interminable hours of demanding problems. I wanted to go home. I'd stormed out after a bad argument with my wife and needed to patch things up by doing justice, for once, to the excellent lunch she always lovingly prepared. I was locking up when the phone rang.

'Dr Veriform,' I said curtly.

'It's the missus,' said Mr Graymouth. Ewan Graymouth. I knew he wouldn't ring me frivolously. I also knew he lived a long way out.

'What seems to be the problem?' I asked, resigned.

'She's right off her food. Can't keep anything down.'

I sighed, I'm afraid with no good grace whatsoever. 'I'll be right there.'

To access the Graymouth farm, I drove into a swampy area 5–6 miles along a narrow windy mountain road. Sharp class distinction existed in southern New Zealand, with cow cockies and sheep cockies comprising the local landed gentry. The farms of some wealthy farmers were worth $250 an acre then, millions now. People round Banded Plover and Mile High were mostly subsistence farmers. Made no difference to me. If they wanted a house call, they got it, rich or poor.

I sped along the road. Generally, I like doing house calls, but sometimes you're caught in the surgery and begrudge going out. One thing that stops you doing house calls, and it shouldn't, is not being paid kilometerage. We were paid one-and-three a mile in New Zealand. In those days, all you got from the government was seven-and-six a patient. We charged three-and-six a patient, which everyone paid in cash, unlike the old system way back in the pre–World War II days when we got ten-and-six a call.

Feeling very aggrieved, I called in on the Graymouths. 'Where is she?' I snarled.

Mr Graymouth was a huge man with a dapper goatee, which he constantly smoothed between thumb and forefinger. His Mephistophelian manner was nicely balanced by his wife's general air of mischievousness. The puckish effect was spoiled by her habit of thrusting her neck forward like a turtle. That day, the slender woman with the pixie face was anything but impish. She'd a nasty case of the flu.

I fixed up Mrs Graymouth and prepared to leave.

'Doctor, I've got something for you,' the farmer said quietly, rubbing his chin like mad. He foraged in the deep freeze and brought forth a completely plucked and cooked goose. 'This is your present for Christmas.'

I felt a foot tall. You'd occasionally find a patient who appreciated what you'd done. Sometimes you'd find your car was running heavy in the back end. You'd wonder why and find that while you were seeing a patient, the spouse had loaded your car with a bag of spuds, or something equally welcome.

Mr Graymouth was one of the grateful ones, with myself in a bad temper and presented with a clean, plucked goose for Christmas.

I slunk out the door.

Perhaps I shouldn't have been so emotional the night a dairy farmer blocked my way on a road long ago in New Zealand. A patient was having a heart attack and it was late. Heavy snow on a straight, 5-mile stretch of road, pitch-black, and an old dairy farmer driving his truck down the middle of the road. I was bound for a sheep cocky in his late 50s who'd been shifting a piano for his wife.

I could not move the old bastard off the road. I blew the horn, to no avail. I was behind him for the best part of 5 miles. It was snowing that nasty, driving stuff, straight from Antarctica, the worst that winter has to offer.

'Bloody farmer won't get off the road and I'm going to an emergency,' I fumed in suppressed fury.

I did *everything* short of running into him. I flashed my lights. I nearly drove up his back end. I blasted the horn. Finally, the old dairyman got the message and veered off to the side. I shot through *heavy* snow at least a foot deep.

I slid to a stop in front of a tidy farmhouse. Like so many others, it was wooden and square with a red galvanised iron roof, a front door in the middle, lounge on the left and three bedrooms on the right. At the end of a long passage were the kitchen and outside loo. The house's exterior was painted creamy white. Inside it was light blue. After the high wool prices of the Korean War, you'd quite often find an old house such as this in the back, say in the pine trees, and a smart new modern house, brick veneer with a tiled roof, in the front. Farmers changed from driving old jalopies to Chevrolet Bel Airs or Mark VII Jaguars.

That night, I bolted round the back after receiving no reply at the front door. The bluish-white blowing cold ended abruptly, replaced by warm rushing yellow. Plump, dairy-fed Mrs Jack opened the door before I applied clenched fist to wood. Ah, the smells, the lingering joy, the deliciousness of a successful roast dinner! Before me arose images of shooting from table to sick patient, reluctantly abandoning many of Olive's meals. I mourned desiccated potato bullets and limp green vegetables.

'Doctor, we expected you sooner.' Mrs Jack was unable to keep the reproach from her voice. She led me across the cosy kitchen that sang out to me to stay.

'So did I,' I blurted irritably. I was immediately sorry. Mrs Jack was upset.

'He's in here.'

She deposited me in the chilly parlour. Mr Dewey Jack was stretched out on the sofa with his clothes on, reinforced with a home-made crocheted quilt. It was one of those glorious creations of squares of unlikely coloured yarn left over from knitting jumpers, scarves and stockings. I ruminated fleetingly on the previous use of a garment that was red shot with silver. It made the poor man look even greyer. He was very sick.

In those days, we relied entirely on our clinical skills. There were no portable ECGs and such. I knew immediately what was wrong. 'You've had a bad heart attack, Mr Jack. You need to be hospitalised.'

I gave the farmer some morphine for the pain.

'Thank you, doctor,' Dewey Jack said.

His wife was equally appreciative.

Patients will thank you if you're heavy-handed with drugs, but none ever expressed gratitude when I trod lightly. We forget that opium and heroin were ingredients in many old concoctions, and efficacious they were for sedation and pain relief. A lovely antidiarrhoeal called Mist. Cret. Aromat. c. Opio moved an elderly farmer to say, 'What was that stuff wot you give me, doctor? It was good for me bowls.' The multidrug culture stopped that, which is a shame. With the opiates, you had morphine in cold syrups. A celebrated one, Dover's Powder, contained opium and ipecacuanha – an emetic – so increasing the dosage caused you to vomit, which was clever. Curious they haven't kept that up. It wasn't a huge problem. It's surprising how late opium was put on the dangerous-drugs register. You could get laudanum, that mixture of opium and alcohol, by going to the chemist and being the right-looking sort of chap. One patient, a chemist, or pharmacist, was hooked on intramuscular adrenalin. He'd steal it and give himself injections. One was cautioned to be conservative in Hong Kong, because nannies put a tiny sliver of opium under their fingernails, which babies sucked; the infants were always terribly well behaved. The tranquilliser of my day was a mixture of amphetamine and barbiturate. I used that a lot. Later, we got a sleeping tablet that allowed patients to down a hundred and not do themselves any harm. It was widely used. It was *wonderful*, was thalidomide. Happily, I never gave it to a pregnant woman – more luck than judgement, I think.

That stormy winter's night, Dewey Jack was duly driven by ambulance to hospital. He recovered quite well in the long run and followed my advice, as far as I know, not to shift large musical instruments.

As a result of that home visit, I met a schoolteacher to whom I later gave away a local Scottish girl in marriage. Two years later, I got to the hospital in plenty of time to deliver their baby, but I'm getting ahead of myself. This man was called Jack Junior because he was the son of my piano-moving patient. Jack Junior was a vintage-car fan. I'd told him at his father's bedside about not being able to blast that dairy farmer off the road and promptly forgotten it. One day 6 months later, I hunched over the table bolting down yet another lunch. As it was Wednesday, I had my maternity girls – my pregnant patients. Dear Olive, who'd long given up admonishing me not to eat so fast, turned from washing dishes at the sink and said casually, 'A parcel's arrived for you from Scotland, dear.'

This was a noteworthy event. 'Bring it to me,' I ordered.

She complied, and hovered over my shoulder.

I opened it without delay. Ensconced in the nested packing material sat an astounding object.

My wife pulled out a card. 'It's from Jack Junior.'

I was moved that the young man remembered me on his honeymoon. From the bottom of the box I plucked an English motoring magazine he'd caringly enclosed and turned to a highlighted article. 'It's a Maserati air-blast horn called *il trombe ultimo*.'

It certainly was the ultimate trumpet. Its circuit was separate from the rest of the car and took so much power that the lights dimmed a few weeks later when I blew the horn to blast another inconsiderate farmer off the road. I've used it successfully on various New Zealand farmers, but not dared set it up elsewhere. The local policeman here assures me that I can install it, but sadly my present Commodore – a nightmare of wires, parts and air-conditioning gear – has no room for Mediterranean masterpieces.

Yes, *il trombe ultimo* worked. It got them off the road all right, but not always the way it should. Two years after *il trombe ultimo* joined us, the phone rang one Sunday morning. It was Mrs Jack. 'Doctor, Josie's in labour,' she said of her daughter-in-law. I heard stress and joy battling in Mrs Jack's voice. A third generation prepared to inhabit the house and she was being crowded out.

'Tell Jack Junior to meet me at the maternity home.'

I drove madly, hoping to attain my destination before the staff delivered another baby without me. I lost our running bet all too often, despite the fighting chance that *il trombe ultimo* gave me. I had not counted on Iris McBride.

Imagine an elderly lady in an even-older car on her way to church, driving down the middle of a narrow country lane quite sedately in broad daylight, encased in an aura of sanctity. Dear old Iris, with her round red face and air of perplexed innocence. She was one of those legions, both wed and unwed, whose easy bruising renders them temperamentally unsuited to the rough and tumble of marital life. Iris lived with her elder sister in a cottage left by their widowed father. She tended her sister with all the devotion of an adored youngest child.

There had been three brothers, two of whom they lost in war. One died in child-hood. Iris' life contracted to encompass her garden bed and tea table. Life's noises were suppressed – no belches or loud quarrels – and life's passions long forgotten. Each time I drank a cup of tea with the sisters on a home visit, I found that Iris had divested herself of another drop of life's juice. Sororal chatter revolved around: 'Have another, Iris.' 'Oh no, I shouldn't.' 'Listen to your elder sister. You know you've always been partial to my shortbread.' 'I couldn't.'

Here I come at 80 miles an hour, like something out of *Mad Max*, in a souped-up car, bearing down on poor Iris, who was doing nineteen, tops. The oblivious Iris continued on her way to commune with her god as if she were taking the car out for a walk. She even patted it fondly.

I hit *il trombe*, determined to win this bet.

Poor Iris! She got such a fright that, instead of pulling over to the left, she veered to the right as I was passing her. I ended up on the wrong side of the road, in the dirt, power poles flashing by – and made it! I think I nearly sent Iris to her maker.

Yes, I arrived at the maternity home in good time. Father and doctor toasted the emergence of Jack Junior's junior. The hospital administrator joined us.

In those days, bureaucrats in New Zealand were different. And in Australia? Olive and I would soon find out.

Locked up in chains

Barker Kaye

'Chains, my baby's got me locked up in chains, and they're the kind that you can't see . . .'

For one home visit, I recall the circumstances leading up to my arrival more than the consultation itself. I envision a boy in chains every time I pass a certain cottage on my way to my bit of bush, with chainsaw, splitter, logging fuels and tools piled in the back of the four-wheel-drive. I'd better tell you how I got my nickname, Barker, to give you a feel for the bush before I launch into this story.

Not long after I bought this place, a logger friend was felling six gum trees: two for me, two for him and two for the sawmiller. That suited me, as the land's purchase price had felled my savings. I was sitting on a freshly barked log, drinking instant coffee from a Thermos cup. Precise names for the different shades of green in the forest meant nothing out here. Jade, olive, chartreuse: how could they compare to the glow of an unfurling fern frond or the blackening of serrated sassafras leaves that splintered the canopy as I squinted into the sun? The scents of city life claimed me during the week, but now, now the forest embraced me for her own. Ah, my first love.

The devotion of my wife couldn't breach my slippery slopes. 'Barker is willin',' I said, proposing marriage. Her blank stare foretold a safe union. Only out here did the separateness leave me, the relentless niggling. In time it engorged with patients, like dear old Mrs B, tubercular Tenpa Dawa in South India and the desolate Allan Pym, doomed to drive away what he needed most.

I nestled the black cup into a pile of rotting twigs, heaved the axe into the tree's cleavage and gave a little push. My rubber-soled boots slid down the balding log. A freshly barked tree was absolutely slippery. Water spurted from the log like a jet under pressure. The healthier the tree, the easier to bark. A tree almost dead at the top required much more time. A 10.2-metre gum like this one took anywhere from 10 minutes to 2 hours, depending on the bark. The average was half an hour. Sawmillers rejected brown trees, which indicated significant bark. These days, they wanted barked trees and passed on the cost to the logger, generating quite an expenditure in labour, not to mention that freshly barked, slick trees were dangerous to winch onto the truck. Bark has many layers, like onion skins and doctors still seeking a niche. That closest to the tree is white.

Tearing little strips made baby peeling sounds. Ripping long strips elicited a deeper, throatier flaying.

Previously, only boys and women barked logs because it was unskilled. Logging is very skilled work. Barking was repetitive and hypnotic, freeing my mind to wander. I appreciated the forest but possessed the luxury of moral and professional choice. I might not be waxing so lyrical if I were unskilled with a family to feed.

The bulldozer engine of my logger friend, Deadeye (he picked within inches where he'd drop his trees), idled as he released the winch rope from a newly felled tree. Clangs accompanied my unhooking of the rope, a heavy steel coil which encircled the log for dragging out behind the 'dozer. Deadeye wore ear-muffs and manoeuvred the bulldozer as if it were a toy. The engine whined and growled as the dozer hauled logs. It bumped out of the forest, blades knocking, and squeaked and thumped its rocking way over bark and new dirt paths.

My labours unshrouded a beetle and a black, lethal-looking insect with mas-sive pincers. The beetle toddled along unthreateningly, but the scorpion-like insect scurried straight for me. I brushed him off with my boot, into a pile of wombat poo and inhaled with relief, sucking up scents of gum trees, sweat and sassafras.

The air was crisp inside a soggy trail of 'dozer diesel. Mosquitoes whined, and bark snuffled on fallen leaves. A sharp crack took a branch to the ground with a muffled thud. Flies buzzed in different pitches, like dive-bombers and harried commuters. Chainsaw and flying sawdust. Axe echo. Crunch underfoot: fallen leaves and dead twigs. Follow the 'dozer's path: tyre tread on bare brown earth.

The scale of life on my land changed things. Standing under a *Eucalyptus viminalis*, 22 feet in circumference and 500 years old, slotted my problems in perspective. Being a doctor was like being a logger or a policeman. You were prepared for anything at any time. Disaster lurked around every corner.

I always craved isolation, away from the demands of the day, be they spousal or professional. A life spent adapting and reconciling wasn't in the cards. Welcome to general practice: adapting the patient to the disease or the disease to the patient or treatment, where the personal meets the scientific.

Driving long distances or odd hours for patients gives me time to think. All sorts of things squelch loose: the patient I'm heading towards, my own problems and those of colleagues. Tommy MacDonald once regaled me with the tale of his locum for a mutual friend. Tommy asked the district nurse to swing by and remove the stitches from an old man's leg, as she was going out in that direction anyway. She was happy to oblige, but was required to fill out papers in nonupli-cate. Nine times! That it saved a sick old man who lived a long way out a lot of bother was inconsequential. Tommy said he'd do it himself.

Driving gives me closure. Hypnotic engine sounds and eucalypti whizzing past, repetitive hand-and-foot movements combined with the requisite alertness sends me into a trance-like state which hooks right into the problem-solving centre of my brain. If I wanted closure, general practice was the worst place to be. Patients flitted through, like those on holiday. Was it bronchitis or something sinister? Did I miss meningitis in that screaming infant? The night in hospital when a young mum brought in her sick baby haunts me. I was exhausted, but that's no excuse. I said to bring him back if he got worse. I pray it wasn't meningitis and that the child's not brain-damaged or dead. I envy those GPs whose families germinate in one location and contentedly offer cradle-to-grave service generation after generation.

Sometimes, home visits raise more questions than they answer and do not always provide closure. Look at poor old Dexter Veriform. He's got himself embroiled in a lethal set of professional chains called femocrat, and he's no Houdini. Some of us doubt he'll be able to survive the sustained attack of that certain sort of paper-pusher who always wins the skirmishes and battles of general practice. I'm a private person and do whatever I can to avoid them, and I plan to keep it that way. I once did a locum for Dexter, and never met a doctor who loved his patients more. They were damned lucky to have him. That offended femocrat had the great misfortune to stumble upon something that should have remained private, between doctor and patient. Please God, don't let that happen to me. May I mollify, bore or be invisible to every bureaucrat I meet.

I confirmed for myself one morning that closure could be elusive, even in post-visit dissection on a ribbon of road with a 1960s girl group singing from the dashboard.

'Will you come, doctor, to the old Brown place?' asked a voice at the end of a telephone. I was relieving a friend for a week, the same friend for whom Tommy McDonald worked, the one with the accommodating nurse. The caller hung up before I got directions. This was before I bought land in the area, so all I knew was to go to a village with a few old weatherboard buildings 15 minutes' drive away.

I set off in my old truck. It turned quickly from one of those sparkling days – with a sky so blue and air so pure the leaves shimmered – to a blustery day with pelting rain. In these days of drought, I miss certain sounds, like rain on the roof and the kerplunk of windscreen wipers across my field of vision. A fast kerplunkkerplunkkerplunk keeps the pounding water away, and a scraping kerrrrplunk dissolves the droplets.

Like many doctors here, my principal chose quality of life over career advancement. He preferred not to use this place as a stepping stone to scale the medical heights, unlike his two ex-partners. They found a legal loophole and slipped in from far-flung *white* corners of the Commonwealth. Their non-Caucasian colleagues worked as slaves indentured to their registration, in either remote rural areas or that infamous hospital where no competent Caucasian ever sets foot.

I pulled off a sealed road into the potholed drive of a weatherboard house, intending to ask directions. I was ready for anything. Or so I thought.

Three images accompanied me as I knocked, wagging fatherly fingers, admonishing me to expect the unanticipated: Zoltan Nagy in his buttery leather loafers, Dexter Veriform in his old car laden with patients' gifts and the spidery Thucydides Hare creating chaos in the kitchen along with his beetroot bread. The unexpected took many forms. I'd long steeled myself against the temptations of flimsy female negligee, but the lonely advances of Mr Pym exposed a moral crack in my medical facade. I wasn't the only doctor caught off-guard. The sudden appearance of bulls and dogs urinating on their car windows surprised one colleague. Tommy MacDonald hit a camel that materialised in front of his car in the desert.

That pale-pink house raised no warning bells. My guard was down, anaesthetised into inaction by the undulating rhythms of the road and the windscreen wipers. I ran to the door through the rain. A slender teenage boy answered my knock. His jeans and T-shirt were clean and freshly pressed. His eyes were clear. Spots dotted his chin. He appeared to be completely normal. Except for one thing.

I could not help but notice the chains round his ankles.

'Sorry to disturb you,' I said politely, ignoring the constraints. 'Where's Mrs Brown's house?'

I was brought up not to discuss strange or painful subjects.

'A little farther, that way.' Leaning and pointing rattled the boy's shackles. He did not appear to be in any pain, so I left.

That was it. One question, one response, and that interlude lingers to this day.

The rain and approaching consultation left me no time to ruminate on unrumpled boys in chains. I understood later, when I moved to the area, that different chains bound my patient to her daughter-in-law. Eighty-eight-year-old Mrs China Brown lived with the rather simple Younger Mrs Brown, as she was known. She was in her 40s, looked 60 and acted 20. They'd lived alone for 13 years, since a logging accident claimed the son/husband. The husband/father-in-law died long ago, before anyone checked for arsenic poisoning. When the son/husband departed, his women simply tidied up the mess left by a widow-making eucalyptus. A more eccentric couple you could not find, with their own way of living carved by years of mutual accommodation.

The two women inhabited a weatherboard house opposite an old stone church in one of those small towns that are all wide main streets flanked by 1950s glass storefronts and angled parking. The village typified this corner of the world, with houses spread round a few bends in a narrow road before dissipating into paddocks full of green grass and creamy Jersey cows.

I fought my way through a solid wall of pounding rain to the Browns' back door. At least I'd be able to dry off once I got inside. An icy finger of water found the gap between my hair and coat collar and trickled down my back.

'Oh, doctor, it's you,' said the quavering voice of Younger Mrs Brown. 'Come in.' Her hair was matted and mouldy, parched with age and rampant with dandruff. 'She aches all over, poor old dear.' The daughter-in-law yanked her head to the side.

I suspected the flu. It was going around.

I'd one arm out of my overcoat when I froze into immobility. The roof leaked in loud drips. The floor was substantially muddy. The kitchen was incredibly messy. Open tins of corn and beetroot sat on the bench top, their lids wrenched partly off. Dirty dinner plates and teacups infested the remaining expanse. What drives one person round the bend, another does not notice. I swallowed, reinserted wet arm into dank coat and threaded through the empty cans of peas and bread packets that littered the carpet. The whole floor was basically mud and rubbish.

The daughter-in-law led me to the old lady, over muck so deep it obscured the boundary between floor and bed.

'What's the problem, Mrs Brown?' I asked, bending over. She smelled damp and smoky.

I treated the elderly lady, left the script, without which they all felt no consultation was complete, and left smartly.

Without doubt, this was the seediest place I've ever been called to, and the smelliest. These two ladies were perfectly content in their chaos, as sometimes occurs with the elderly, mentally incapable and depressed: a slide into squalor that often ended in death or incarceration in a nursing home. My sister should send my 15-year-old nephew to live with the Browns. He'd feel right at home. But patients surprised one, and people sometimes rocketed out of their filth into immaculacy.

I negotiated the winding drive home with the chained teenager fluttering at mind's edge. Was he in trouble? Should I have said or done something? My upbringing failed me again. That set off a whole new chain of ruminations.

I had to confirm that he was okay, so I turned off the road into his driveway and grabbed my medical bag. The sun was out, giving a pearly tint to the house's pink paint. I rang the bell, not knowing what to expect. That was years ago, before escalating violence against doctors. These days, I'm not so sure I'd have retraced my steps.

The same boy answered, this time unhobbled. He swung a half-full beer bottle nervously from one hand.

'Excuse me,' I said with a combination of sensitivity and authority, 'My name is Dr Kaye. When I stopped to ask directions before, there were chains round your ankles.'

'Oh,' he said with a dismissive wave of the beer bottle, 'I was just playing a game.'

'I see.'

I stood for a while. Neither of us said anything.

'Are you all right?'

'Yeah.'

'You're certain?'

'Yeah, yeah.'

'Well, call me if you need me and I'll come out.'

He grunted.

I'd no reason for me to stay, so I left. I think of him whenever I pass, on the way to my land in the bush.

The teaberry patch in Doctors Bog

Petra Neumann

I was a lot smarter than my four brothers, but my parents sent them to university and told me there wasn't enough money – I'd need a scholarship if I wanted to do medicine. I worked part-time, and it all overwhelmed me. I dropped out and became a psychologist, which gave me breathing space to recover from exhaustion. But it wasn't what I really wanted. I'd *settled*. It ate away at me. Reading medical fiction drove me back into the arms of my beloved profession, where I've nestled happily ever since.

They say we're more liberal in the West. Dr Manning, one of my instructors at medical school, worked in Iraq in the 1950s. If a middle-class daughter was smarter than her brothers, she was the one the family sent to university. My brothers squeaked through with commerce degrees and became financial planners. Hah. I'd not trust them with my hard-earned pennies. Dr Manning found the Bedouins free and easy; women were promiscuous within their own tribe and didn't wear the veil. Once, he was smuggled into Syria to examine the eight-month-old baby of a customs official. He diagnosed FTT: failure to thrive. No one could work it out. The family lived in a nice, clean mud-brick house. Dr Manning examined the baby and the mother and found nothing wrong. He was thinking fast and hard at that point. Suddenly, little five-year-old Ali ran in and took a breast. As the mother hailed from a remote village far away, she'd no older female relatives to aid in child-rearing and explain not to breastfeed the five-year-old when there was a newborn. Dr Manning left some nutritional supplement drops, because they liked to have something in hand, and explained to the mother through an interpreter the necessity of weaning Ali.

I wished I'd weaned my own son the time we attended the stabbing. I was gone all day and ended up leaking down my shirt and trousers. My senior partner, Charles, was mortified.

First let me tell you how I met my husband. I'd been called out to the Nesbitts, a thirty-something couple originally from Britain who personified the restless searching for Enough Time that plagues our generation. They jumped off the rat's wheel, forsook the race to pursue the important things of life. All this free time brought them face to face with something they were unprepared and unwilling to address. The Nesbitts' escape from the humdrum had used up their allotment of courage. They'd none left for the rocky journey. Subsequently, Jimmy compressed his desperation into narrowed eyes, grim mouth and jutting chin that accentuated the turmoil within. The volcano of Fiona's disillusion erupted in fiery words that scorched all in her path. 'Iceberg' may be a better metaphor, as Fiona hid so much beneath water level that speared the unsuspecting. Jimmy piloted the ferry back and forth and performed the numerous manly chores expected in the islands. At the end of the day, he was too tired for self-expression through the fine art of painting. Fiona was fortunate that she could practice singing anytime, much to Jimmy's annoyance. Another little tug on the heartstrings tautened his mouth and eyes. And Fiona's knife-tongue slashed: he wasn't much of a provider, after all, was he, forcing her to work too bloody hard. Wrong thing to say to a short man.

A male voice rang the clinic one morning at teatime. 'Our daughter fell from her pony.' Jimmy ran me over to a one-family island. The woman of the house took me back to the house, filling me in as we walked. We'd got as far as the kitchen when a muffled voice said, 'I know what the problem is.' All that was visible was a corkscrewed swathe of strong back with its head in the heater.

'That's Alec, fitting new bricks in the firebox,' the mother said, pointing at the wood heater. 'I'll get Jimmy. He's got to eat, too.'

I made for the bedroom.

'Stay for dinner, won't you, doctor?' she asked, speaking in sparks. 'You and Alec.' She waved a carving knife at the figure emerging from the heater's depths and pointed it in the direction of the stove. 'Only three-six-five and spuds.'

I accepted the invitation to dinner, as they called the midday meal. 'Three-six-five' meant mutton, which they ate from Monday to Sunday. Spuds must have run a close second: I ate them boiled, baked, mashed, fried, hot and cold, with butter, cream, three-six-five gravy and with onions, eggs and tomato sauce.

As Nora Ephron said in the film *Heartburn*, 'I have made a lot of mistakes falling in love, and regretted most of them, but never the potatoes that went with them.' I didn't regret Alec Porter, not for a minute, not even in my darker moments.

I treated the girl for greenstick fracture – so common in children. They'd already begun to eat by the time I made it to the dining table. The son of the house was off somewhere, and the girl wasn't hungry. Five adults sat on wooden benches at a sturdy hand-made table.

Here's love encapsulated, island-style: 'This is Alec Porter. He's not married, and he's the right age for you.' Fiona Nesbitt pointed a fork at a tall man totally devoid of body hair, who paused in the act of shovelling potatoes into his mouth to nod at me. It gave me a jolt to be treated like a farm animal. Women marry and breed here, and that's that.

'Have some spuds,' said he, pausing in mid-scoop to slide the steaming bowl my way.

'Don't tip them over,' Fiona said.

One thing led to another, and I ended up declaring at my wedding that Alec was the only man for me, stating it with a vehemence I might not have felt in the city, with enough women to go around. I squirmed at the need I saw reflected in men's eyes and the exhaustion in women's.

Was it really love? I was probably slumming if I'm totally honest, avoiding an appropriate relationship. Timing is so important. I knew the biological clock was ticking. Alec's and my backgrounds were too different. But ah, it was sweet while it lasted.

I carried on working after my marriage. Amaranth Fillet appeared a week before I delivered my son, thankfully. Her competence gave me a treasured break. Sadly, her own drummer marched her away too soon. We got in another locum because I insisted on not working until my baby was 12 weeks old, but this fly-by-night practitioner was hopeless on horseback, which made him useless to me. I'm probably being too hard on him, but his intractability irritated me.

Now I've shepherded us through my reasons for seeking such remoteness, my marriage and my child, and brought us to 10 weeks after Ronnie's birth. I found myself on horseback early one morning during shearing season to attend an attempted murder. The settlement manager and our pilot accompanied Charles and me through Doctors Bog. Mrs McShane claimed the best teaberry patch on the islands was 'a-ways in there.' She used it for her jam. The jar she'd given me after the condom episode came from this patch. I needed to breastfeed my son and resented being recalled from leave because our locum was not up to this. I focused on Alec and Ronald. How was my baby doing without my milk? How was my husband doing with the infant? Stabbings and other emergencies were not unheard of at this time of year; perhaps I should put together a stock of expressed milk.

'Why is it called Doctors Bog?' I asked, surly.

'Oh, we've lost a few,' the manager replied casually.

'What, doctors?'

'Yeah.'

'Did you get them out?'

The omnipresent loch magnified everything in sight. We rose along the magenta- and plum-coloured moor. Heavy summer rain intensified the heather. Midges and clegs competed with wind and water for airspace. I swatted and swiped. Mist bathed us in droplets that consolidated a pointillist painting. Somewhere in the distance, a waterfall cymballed and rolled.

'Did we get them out? The horses, no; the doctors, mostly.'

The 'mostly' rode beside me in the form of a doctor who would always survive, carried by the quiet bay to a migrant worker stabbed in a brawl, in what would become the first murder of the century, and it was the 1990s.

Fortunately, the journey was short, 2 hours each way, not the nightmare endured by my predecessor. The poor man spent 48 hours by horseback for what was normally a 13-hour ride to attend a child with suspected appendicitis. Four men lifted him off the horse and carried him to the Big House. Two days of intensive nursing got his joints moving sufficiently to examine the child, who'd since recovered. My predecessor left soon after.

During that time, I considered giving my son cow's milk. I doubted he'd accept it. Our dairy was simply a guy who milked a few cows. He ladled milk out of a huge great crate into itch-cream bottles, tomato sauce bottles, vodka bottles, scotch bottles – whatever was available. You recognised people's tipples by what was left full of milk at the back door.

'He's round the back,' said the manager as we approached the house. 'We all know who did it, but we can't prove it.'

Charles and I knelt down in the dirt, by the back door. I folded back the blanket, whose wool smelled musty and scratched my fingers. My senior partner pulled away bits of rough cotton shirt.

'The knife has split the stomach open,' Charles said. His guts were hanging out and stuck with peat. 'We'll have to anaesthetise him and sew him up.' Turning to the manager he said, 'He needs to be inside and on the kitchen table.'

'Right.'

'And we'll need some hot water. A lot of it.'

A momentary hesitation revealed the manager's resentment of an interruption to the important shearing by an expendable peon.

After some door banging and table scraping as patient and operating equipment were manoeuvred into position, Charles and I set to the task at hand. We worked fast, but the patient started to deteriorate.

'He's bleeding!' I said, searching for the bleeding vessel to tie off.

'We'll have to stabilise him enough to get him out of here,' Charles said.

After accomplishing that feat, we rethreaded through Doctors Bog with the patient on a stretcher between two horses. My breasts started to leak as we passed Mrs McShane's teaberry bushes on the way to the boat.

When we got back, we proceeded straight to theatre. By this time, it was 7:00 at night. Now remember, my 10-week-old baby was totally breastfed. I was standing in greens with milk coursing down and filling up my white theatre boots.

Charles – o disbeliever in birth control – was too embarrassed to eyeball me.

The migrant worker was not salvageable at the end of the day. We lost him.

The whole house was in darkness when I got home, except for one little light in the sitting room. The car was out front, so I knew that my husband was home. Not a sound could be heard anywhere. I looked in the bedroom. Nobody. I heard a weak, scratchy 'Aha-aahhh-ahhh' in the bathroom down the hall.

My husband was lying in the bath, water up to his neck. He rocked our son on his chest with his head poking from the water. Ronald hadn't stopped screaming for hours. Alec took him to hospital. He refused every bottle. The only way to keep him quiet and contented was in the bath. Both husband and son were wrinkly around the edges.

When we got it all sorted out, my husband said, 'Don't ever do that again.'

That was all that was said.

I made sure Alec used our abundant supply of condoms. He wanted more children, a whole bunkhouse of farmhands. Not likely. He wanted home-cooked meals and teas, five times a day, but I wasn't a cottage cat. He knew that when he married me, but he hoped I'd change, as he spat out in many many a frustrated moment. I was torn. It was only a matter of time until I left the islands. I wanted to pack up my son, but couldn't wrench Ronald from his father and his home. I've not been able to convey that sense of place to my urban friends and colleagues, that feeling of amputation. My son's arteries and veins were the islands' trees, his blood its water. For years, I debated, ossifying into inaction. Going out to little Annie Hart presented me with a solution, perhaps imperfect but nonetheless the best I could do.

Ronald crawled, toddled and ran after his father into the peat. His first job was to carry the pocketknife, which he performed with all the artless resolution of a young son determined to please his father. Like all island men, my husband was breathtakingly self-sufficient, except for one little problem: he was absent-minded. He was always losing his pocketknife, which was a big thing. 'I accidentally drowned it, doctor.' 'The dog buried it.' 'I left it out overnight and a wolf got it.' Wolf? He was always waiting for a new one on the supply ship. The women fussed over him and the men tittered.

From the time little Ronnie was able to carry it, no pocketknives met unpleasant fates. I couldn't leave the boy or extract him from the man and the land. I ensured that he received a good education, in the local school and at home. And so life continued for some years, and before I knew it, Ronald was 9 years old, like Annie Hart.

We picked up the little girl in a plane called a Beaver. This bush plane has STOL – short takeoff and landing – and can be fitted easily with wheels, floats or skis, so it's ideal in remote and rugged areas. We used it all the time.

Annie and her family lived way, way out, on one of the farthest single-family islands. We treated these people warily. Their extreme isolation corroded their interactive skills.

Annie was the ruddy kind of blonde with rude health, not the pale sort with skin so translucent the veins danced. The Harts' diet was adequate. Mutton and spuds was the dinner staple. Women milked cows that produced copious amounts of milk and cream and beautiful home-made butter. They ate cream cakes for morning tea, cold meat and cream for lunch and scones with cream for afternoon tea. They ended the day with cream-on-something. They seemed reasonably healthy despite a high-fat diet. Annie's great-grandfather was 87 and still on horseback, rounding up sheep and cutting his own peat.

Annie's mother ran to meet us when the pilot landed the Beaver on the water. This was a special occasion, so she changed into a dress. It was made from an old flour sack, but it was quite pretty.

'She's up in the house, doctor,' Mrs Hart said, jerking her head towards a stream of peat smoke rising over a dip in the cliff.

I love the sharp scent of peat, so different from city smells like engine exhaust. Most island men cut a tonne of peat in the morning before they leave for work. It was hard on backs.

'She's not saying much, but I know she's in pain,' Mrs Hart said slowly.

'What happened?'

'I was pegging out the wash and saw her roll down the side of a cliff. Annie thinks she's a bird, and sometimes she looks like one. Her feet hardly touch the ground when she's on them cliffs.'

I'd a job to keep up with Mrs Hart as she strode to a typical farmhouse, with galvanised iron roof and sheeting. Some houses on the islands were stone. A very very few were made of wood. Occasionally, somebody imported bricks, but they were expensive.

Inside, the house was wood-panelled halfway up, with plasterboard above that. The kitchen was plain wood. It was quite large, and included a sitting room/living area. A big combustion stove ran on peat. The Harts' colour scheme was amazing, entirely in keeping with the casual attitudes of the islanders. The outside was plain, but inside, well, they'd started with orange paint, run out and finished with red. This creative use of colour schemes continued through a bathroom and three bedrooms (away from the heat and quite cold), and what they called the pantry out the back. Not many people owned fridges and deep freezes, since the maximum temperature in summer was only around 13°C. Meat was kept in a dedicated safe out the back door. The laundry was separate from the house, with a twin tub that ran off the generators. They reserved the formal sitting room for visitors, feast days, weddings and birthdays.

'She's in the sitting room, doctor,' Mrs Hart called over her shoulder as she strode through the kitchen.

Annie exhibited typical stoicism. She lay quietly, elbow bent, in her shirt, trackpants, tennis shoes and hand-knitted jumper.

'Annie, the doctor's here to have a look at you,' Mrs Hart said.

'No!' Annie cried, pulling away her arm as I examined it.

One look at that bruised and swollen elbow told me she had a compound fracture.

'What happened, Annie?' I asked gently, wanting to hear her version.

'I slipped up,' she said.

'I'm always telling her to be careful,' said her mother.

'I'm all right,' Annie insisted.

'Annie, your elbow is broken. I'd like to take you back and fix it up properly.'

'I'll carry her,' said her mother.

'I can walk, Mum!' She tried to stand.

I restrained her. 'You can't do it alone, Annie,' I said. 'First, you'll need something for the pain.' I prepared an injection of pethidine. 'The ride may be choppy.'

'We going in the yellow Beaver?' she asked.

'Yes.'

'Um,' she replied, with an impenetrable expression.

The child and I were soon airborne. She was quite nervous.

'Ever been in a plane before?' I asked.

She shook her head.

I held her hand. That humble act often helps more patients than stethoscope and lancet. We passed the plane's hangar on our left as we flew into the capital and landed on the water.

Suddenly, Annie erupted. 'Jesuuus Chriiist!'

'What's the matter?' I cried. Had something gone horribly wrong?

She was quite agitated. Pointing to our left, she cried, 'Two bloody Beavers!' It never occurred to her we'd have more than one plane. To be in one aircraft and spot another nearly undid her.

I settled the child. We were both deeply rattled. Annie and Ronald were friends. She was my son's future. How could I reveal to him other aspects of life without disturbing the father–son relationship or wrenching him from the land he loved? My only solution was to face the demons awakened by Mr Kenneth Dean and provide an alternative lifestyle for my nine-year-old. He might never want it – he hasn't so far – but he'd be exposed to the outside world.

We fixed Annie up and sent her home as soon as we could. Unfortunately, an emergency near Doctors Bog prevented my accompanying Annie's return to her island.

Subsequently, people became less isolated and self-sufficient. Society changed, but that's another story.

Time drained the colour and juice from Ken Dean's threats, so I returned to my old practice after 12 years away. The night before I left, I dreamed that on my first day back at work, the receptionist handed me an envelope with 'Private and Confidential' spiking across the lower left in red. I tore it open and unfolded a piece of copybook paper. My fingers trembled as I read, 'You're back. So am I.' Colour flooded those dark memories, which soon rehydrated themselves and emerged juicy into consciousness in the form of the long-ago home visit which changed my career trajectory and my life. Certifying Ken Dean sent me fleeing to the remotest place I could find, and now I was going back. Was it courageous, weak, foolhardy or desperate? Was I *really* doing it for my child's education, or was I propelled – compelled – by that morbid fascination in which one is drawn to what one wishes to avoid?

Putting down pooch

David Snow

I've always viewed euthanasia as a slippery slope to putting down Grandma or Cousin Mike, who wasn't quite right. I did it once, to a patient's dog. Never again. I mean that. But now our own aged German shepherd is suffering, and what should I do? I don't know. I just don't know. To begin at the beginning.

Huffing up the mountain got a little harder each Christmas, for myself and the children's German shepherd, who always accompanied me. We called him Pimpant – French for smart and natty, one of my kids was studying the language at the time – after a well-dressed patient who'd presented him as a gift. Both doctor and dog were glad we'd exerted ourselves when we reached the summit. The view put the year in perspective. People wander in and out of mining towns, families on the dole looking for cheap housing, doctors on the run, tourists poking through the mine museum, noses in guidebooks or necks craned high at the murals. A tourist and a miner stand out.

Our family called my tourist patient Pimpant Père because he was the father of our dog. Soon we were calling him Perry Pimpant. Anyone who's owned a German shepherd knows the breed is afflicted with hip dysplasia, of whose ramifications we were blissfully ignorant when the irresistible puppy bounded into our lives. One lick and that was that. We kept the dog. The little boy is now preparing to go to university. The dog is limping and his hip catches. He did it hard, huffing up the hill on our annual Christmas outing to our favourite lookout. The vet says his days are numbered.

It began late one Monday afternoon, when a nurse rang from the hospital. 'I've got this guy with something up his bum.'

In medicine, when you want a little time to think, you order an X-ray and hope to come up with something during that process. So I said to myself, 'I suppose you can order an X-ray on a vibrator, depending how far up it is.' I said to the nurse, 'Send him to the surgery.'

'Me and my girlfriend were playing around and put it in,' said Perry the spiffily attired.

'Well, lie down and I'll put me finger up your bum and try to find it.' I felt the rim. I could do it with forceps.

'Right. You go up to the hospital and they'll give you an injection of pethidine. I'll come up and remove it for you.' Which I did half an hour later. He was lying on his side with his legs up. I used long forceps, fiddled around and finally got a hold of this thing.

He was going 'Ooh, ooh, ooh, ooh.' It was that painful.

Obviously, if something's stuck up your bum, you're going to put up with a fair bit. I pulled and pulled, and it finally came out with this great big suction *smack*. I looked at the thing and handed it to one of the nursing sisters, who sniffed it and pronounced what we knew, that it was a big brown plastic doorstopper.

The following day, I asked my receptionist, 'Where's me doorstopper?' I wanted to keep it as a souvenir.

'I sent it down for histology,' she said.

'You what?!'

'I sent it to town.'

I said, 'Ring 'em up and tell 'em I want my doorstopper *back*.'

Turns out they tossed my doorstopper, so someone at the lab scoured hardware shops for half a day. They sent it back with this beautiful histology report, saying how big it was, how long it was, how wide it was, what its diameter was and in conclusion, this is a doorstopper. They included an article on foreign bodies removed from rectums from the Royal Perth Hospital. In 25 of 27 cases, the foreign body was removed under general anaesthetic. When you come out here to our Wild West town, don't expect a general anaesthetic to remove a foreign body from your rectum.

I'd said to this guy, a tourist from the state's capital, 'Come back and see me.' I gave him a date, never expecting him to return, but he did, gift in hand.

'Something for you, doctor,' he said, shyly proffering a German shepherd puppy.

'Not necessary.'

'I wanted to you have him. My sister's dog had puppies. I don't suppose you'd get many cases like mine?'

'You're right, mate, you're the first.' But I don't reckon it was his girlfriend that jammed it up, I reckon it was his boyfriend. Young guy in his 30s, embarrassed, a working-class guy, can't remember how he made a living, but it was nothing spectacular.

And so Pimpant joined the family.

Cyril Johanssen chipped away underground for a quarter-century as times changed overhead. Men and their moods didn't occupy his mind. Cyril Johanssen inched along in incremental unconcern – pick, pick, pick – as the bosses overhead slid to oily irresponsibility for their workers. Claimed we didn't live in a mining town, but a town with a mine in it. Hack, hack, hack. Smooth respect to raggedy greed.

Cyril Johanssen had finished with rolling and roaming and big movements. He underscored this in an act of the sea, by being disgorged on our shore one morning in winter. The loner forsook events on the earth's surface and came to an edge. The edge. Nothing. Mattered. Except. One. Thing. His dog, Kip.

I knew about earth's-end-as-magnet, animal love and responsibility. The journey was a gnawing yearn which everybody here placated with different offerings. The love, well, I had my boys now. I couldn't deny them anything. Like a dog.

One Saturday afternoon outside football season, two metal wheels – miner and medico, weeper and reaper – spun out and skidded. Responsibility marked us forever. To loved ones. To patients.

I'd taken Pimpant, the children's German shepherd, for a stroll. Huffing up the mountain was getting harder for both of us. We were resting when the mobile phone jangled.

'Yeah.'

Oh, no.

'Okay.'

Oh, no.

'I'll meet Cyril at the surgery in about an hour. Don't know if I'll do what he wants, but send him down anyway and we'll see.'

I clicked the phone case shut and turned from the pitted peaks punching into a lunar distance. 'C'mon, boy. Going down'll be easier.'

And it was, but walking alone across to the surgery gave me a ba-a-a-d feeling. Men. Dogs. Boys. Dogs. Soulmates. Pain.

A glance at Cyril's file telescoped his 30-year medical history. A mongrel puppy found him when he retired from the mine after 15 years. My predecessor never minded that the old miner brought Kip to the surgery: 'It amuses the children and makes Cyril happy, so why not?'

Why not, Round Two. What was right became sinister. Something would be left behind shortly that would pit the earth-edge lunar hills in perpetuity.

The bell above the surgery door tinkled, its feathers of sound too insubstantial a scaffolding for the drama about to be erected. Bring on the gongs. Organ. Ding dong avine calling. In jerked a tough old bird with a miner's body: compact and low to the ground, nuggety, so he wasn't always bumping his knees and head on rock faces. No gravity pulled Cyril forward, despite all those years spent eroding earth from inside. Only one thing rounded those shoulders: the load he bore like an offering, forearms extended and parallel, palms cupped. He wept over his mutt, silently, except for the odd uncontainable squawk.

What had I been thinking? I must be mad.

We went into the treatment room and arranged his burden — not that the old miner saw it as such — on the examining table. Cyril murmured and caressed, broken-hearted.

'Doc, I finally decided.' He looked away, eyes streaming. 'Kip's so crippled up with arthritis he can't move on his own anymore. It's time. Could you help us out? Please?' He barked the last word so brutally I nearly started bawling myself.

'Why not take him to the vet?' I was more brusque than I had intended.

'No, we want you to do it.'

'I don't know, Cyril.'

'He trusts you.'

'I've never had a dog as a patient before.'

I thought of Pimpant's worsening hip dysplasia and wondered when this awful dilemma would clamp its iron claw on our family's shoulder.

'Kip's all I got.' Cyril's lower jaw protruded in that belligerent, bulldog way of old east Londoners.

'I'll see what the vet has to say, but no promises, mate.'

The old man pulled at his white hair. It grew over his forehead like a peninsula and emphasised the bullet shape of his head. A .22.

I rang my animal colleague. Punch, punch, punch. 'How do I put down a dog? I've never done it before.' It couldn't be that hard.

It was. Canine anatomy is totally different from ours. You give the dog a big dose of general anaesthetic, and he just goes to sleep. Ideally. You try to get it intravenously, but if you can't you go for intraperitoneally, into the abdomen, but that's more painful.

Together, we positioned the ancient animal. The old miner's arms were shaking. Mine could've been steadier.

The dog gazed up at his master in that way they do, with all that love and trust. Did he know what was coming? I hoped not.

Cyril held Kip the whole time, whispering words I'd rather not repeat. That's between a man and his maker. Or his dog.

I prepared a syringe of diazepam and tried to find Kip's vein. It was harder than I thought. 'Hold him still, Cyril, and keep stroking him like that.'

A terrible sob was my answer. The old man was no longer able to contain the emotional tide.

'Cyril, get a grip! It's not good for him to hear that.' Best not to ponder to whom I was referring. I didn't know how long my own eyes would stay dry.

I couldn't find a vein. 'You can change your mind at any time, Cyril.'

'No, no.'

I started to perspire. 'I'm happy to stop.'

'Just do it, doc!'

I tried again.

The dog started whimpering. *Eee eee eee eee eee.*

Tried again.

Eee eee eee eee eee.

And again.

My eyes blurred. 'I'll have to do it into the abdomen.'

'I don't care, doc. Get it over with.'

So that's what I did.

'I remember when I first got him, doc. He was such a little mongrel. It was love at first sight.'

I swallowed hard, recalling the day Pimpant bounded into our lives. You try telling your child that he cannot have the puppy he's embracing with all the love of which a six-year-old is capable. We kept the dog. That was 12 years ago.

For five long bloody minutes, that dog went *Eee eee eee eee eee.*

The yelps grew softer – the canine ones, that is. Kip died in pain.

'Can I give you something, Cyril?'

'No, no, I got work to do. I'm takin' 'im home with me. He's going out the back.'

I didn't want to know how the miner's tired body could carve out a grave from the grey scree behind his shack. I wanted the corpse off my hands.

I went home and yapped at the kids for making too much noise and almost kicked the dog.

I'll never do that again. I mean it. When people ask me to put down their animals, I send them to Cyril Johanssen, who's done a total volte-face. God knows what the poor man suffered during the 2 months nobody saw him. Whatever it was turned his heart. When his grief released him – or he entered the next phase – Cyril bought a .22 and set himself up as an animal liberator, saying it's quicker and more humane to put a bullet through their heads. Perhaps he's right.

But that's not quite the end of the story. The old miner hates me now. Should I have acted differently? Would Cyril still go to the other doctor and cross the street to avoid me if I'd refused to put down his dog?

Now Pimpant's hip dysplasia is so bad he drags his hind legs.

And I'm dragging my feet.

Gimme that old-time religion ▬▬▬

Nicky Doulton-Brown

Surely my daughter won't be in the mall too much longer. I'm beginning to feel positively sacrificial. I'll distract myself by watching the shoppers. Beautiful women all, well, most. Head coverings can be most attractive, but not those scarves that far-right Christian sect wear. Poor Mrs Black. They made her suffer terribly. Never understood how not seeing your excommunicated brother at the end was the right thing.

I've found that patients with some sort of belief system, not necessarily an organised religion, fare better in times of crisis. It doesn't matter if they believe that God is a cantaloupe or jogging will get them to heaven. Anything will do. There are exceptions, heartbreaking ones, as poor Mrs Black discovered during the last stages of renal failure.

Not everyone conceives of religion as comfort. Some insist that suffering benefits the soul. One thing I hate is to have my patients penalised by the beliefs of their relatives. I'm on dangerous ground. A doctor's role is not to judge his patients or their loved ones, although we're only human. Approbation arises and yes, revulsion. I've learned to keep quiet rather than offend. Nothing wrong with having religion as long as people treat each other well and don't exclude the rest of humanity or require blood sacrifices. One sect got my goat.

They were exclusive. Were they ever. I've always been impressed by what Christian compassion achieves in the world and how it relieves physical suffering, despite the attached proselytising strings of which I disapprove in any religion. I've always felt Christianity's superiority over other faiths is precisely because of this compassion in action. Its sublime art and music enrich our pedestrian world. The Lord was onto a good thing. How did he spawn this particular sect of bigots whose members interpreted the Bible so literally?

It began when a colleague got peeved at climbing a steep hill to sound an old chap's chest first thing in the morning. Probably, it was the first signs of the old doctor's angina. He retired, and I acquired an enormous practice of this Christian sect, who I suspected came to me because as an atheist I was beyond the pale anyway, so no threat.

One morning upon arriving at work, I found my senior colleague hunched over the table in the tearoom, looking grey.

'Are you all right?'

He shook his head. 'This has to be my last time up that mountain. You've recently moved into that old Heritage-listed house down the hill from Mr Wing, I understand.'

'That's right, and I'm happy to take him and his family off your hands, doctor.'

They lived a few blocks from Mrs Dymphna O'Reilly and her neighbours. Mr Wing, Mrs Black and their third sibling, Jamie, found religion after their parents died in an automobile accident. The children were in their teens when a drunken reveller failed to negotiate a corner one night on that winding bit of road heading out of town and hit their parents' car head-on.

It wasn't strictly true that the teenagers found religion; rather, religion found them in their time of grief, in the form of a distant cousin and the sect in question. I hope it gave them solace.

These days, the household consisted of Mr Reginald Wing, his sister, Winifred, and his son, George. They lived in the house in which they were born. Mr Black, my patient's husband, was consigned to the mists of obscurity, a not-uncommon phenomenon in that sect. The third Wing sibling, a university lecturer, was excommunicated years before. The sect's local leader refused any contact between Jamie and his brother and sister.

Reggie Wing moved back home when his wife died. He found George a tremendous burden. As an idealistic young man, he went bush to replicate Thoreau's experiment and laid his treasures at the feet of the sister of a back-woods logger. I realise the implication is offensive. I know dynamic logging contractors who produce quite intelligent children. This family wasn't one of them, being notorious for incest and its consequences. Reggie's wife died young, possibly of a genetic disease which no one got close enough to monitor, leaving only the one child. George was 30 years old at that time.

Curtains rippled in the front window as I relatched the gate and scooted down the walk to the sounds of a scratchy old version of 'The Northern Lights of Old Aberdeen.' Mrs Black led me inside, into the parlour, pulling her scarf close over her ears, and sat near her brother, who was in a wheelchair. George was playing his squeeze box and stamping the floor, which caused the needle to jump on the recording. This didn't stop him from playing along out of tune and out of rhythm. One of the sect's few positive attributes was the soul-searching required of the sect's leaders that resulted in the decision to allow George to keep his squeeze box and record player.

George's stamping was actually quite delicate, considering his build. Generations of solidly built logging-genes-turned-to-fat moved this foot up and down. After a minute, I shouted, 'All right now, Georgie. I'll talk to your dad and we can play hide-and-seek after.'

'Okay,' he yelled back, obediently silencing his squeeze box.

'Why don't you get ready?'

He flashed a toothy smile and trotted off.

'Mr Wing,' I said to the man facing me. He'd have been well over 6 feet in his youth, well suited to his love of playing football for the local team. His health was not good. He'd been so addicted to tobacco he smoked his legs off and the rest of his body into a wheelchair. Mrs Black installed a series of pulleys and chains around the house for him to manoeuvre his chair. I wasn't sure the ceiling was strong enough, but it held. Reggie's most obvious problem was that his dentures made his Ss painfully sibilant, so he whistled when he spoke them.

He nodded slowly. 'You gonna sssound my chessst today, doctor?'

I started doing certain things during an examination that were clinically useless but made people happy every time. No consultation here was complete unless I clapped a stethoscope on what a GP friend called 'scruffy's triangle.' Pull a few shirt buttons open, expose a small wedge near the throat and poke in your stethoscope to do the ritualistic sssounding of the chessst. I obliged. This allowed me to keep an eye on all the members of that household without causing them the insurmountable inconvenience of coming to the surgery. Mr Wing was unable, his son incapable and his sister on the wrong side of the downhill slope of renal problems. I pretended to be engrossed in examining scruffy's triangle as I looked down at Mrs Black's feet. I was checking for oedema under her skirt line. Her ankles and feet weren't too swollen that day.

Mr Wing saw me glance at a framed old photograph on the table. Someone had ripped it, leaving a violent jagged edge in a home filled with love.

'That's me and Winnie in the old days,' Mr Wing said. Like many battlers, he'd aged quickly and appeared to be 20 years older than his 54 winters. He swallowed hard as he pointed to the severed, missing image, a phantom limb that still caused pain. 'That torn-out bit wasss our brother.'

'Is,' interjected Mrs Black softly.

'We're not allowed to have him in the houssse,' Mr Wing explained.

'Will you have a cup of tea, doctor?' Mrs Black asked.

'He doesn't have time, Winnie,' Mr Wing said.

'Sadly, you're right, Mr Wing,' I said. 'No time today, I'm afraid.' Remarkably few folk offer me a cup of tea or a coffee now, and I nearly always have to refuse when they do. I can squeeze in another patient in the time it takes my hot drink to cool enough to consume. 'How are you today, Mrs Black?'

'Very tired, doctor.'

I touched her hand, not only in sympathy but also to check the quality of her skin, which was particular to sufferers of renal disease. She had that distinctive colour.

'Still losing weight?' That much was obvious.

'I'm afraid so. I feel so nauseous.'

'Diarrhoea?'

She nodded. 'I feel a bit better than last week, though' she said, willing it to be so. We were managing her Bright's disease as best we could.

'I'd like to take your blood pressure today.'

'Certainly, doctor.'

It wasn't too bad. After I finished stuffing the cuff into my bag, I asked, 'How's George?'

Brother and sister smiled. Mr Wing named George after his favourite country singer, George Jones. Subsequently, I met other patients named after crooners and television characters, children called Waylon and MacGyver, Madonna and Beyoncé. At least Mr Wing didn't name his son Dolly or Sue.

George loved music, a gene he inherited from his father's side. Winifred

Black studied to be a concert pianist in her youth. Her parents' deaths and the ascendance of the religious cousin put an end to that. George particularly adored Scottish tunes. When I appeared, he pulled out his squeeze box and put the Jimmy Shand & His Band version of 'The Northern Lights of Old Aberdeen' on the turntable. No one cared that he could not play the instrument. Georgie peeked through the curtains when I was due. As soon as he spied me coming down the walk, on popped the gramophone with this old 78-rpm of 'The Northern Lights' – crackle, crackle, needle jump – ''berdeen.' He played it so much the recording was thin as onion skin.

'Time for our game, doc. I bet you can't find me,' George called, pinpointing his exact location.

I tiptoed exaggeratedly to the hallway, saying, 'Now, I wonder where on earth he can be.' The only books the sect allowed were displayed in the bookcases, rows of red, blue and green leather-bound religious tracts written by their boss-man in America. They were forbidden to travel anywhere except on church or medical business, so a number of them contrived to go to the Mayo Clinic in New York when they wanted a holiday.

They didn't have radios or television or insure anything. They relied on their community in times of distress.

I peered past a bookshelf and round the door of Mrs Black's bedroom, waiting for Georgie to spot me. While I waited, a book caught my eye.

'Don't know how interesting you'll find *that*, doctor,' Mrs Black said. She'd slipped in unobserved.

'Don't you miss literature and fine music?'

She sighed. 'Yes, but I'll never accept not being able to contact our other brother. I miss him terribly. We all do.' He'd been flung out long ago for marrying someone outside the church. 'Our cousin won't allow it, and I daren't disobey her.'

That formidably pious creature attended our practice. Before I disgorged my views on the subject of religion as discomfort, Georgie cried out, as always, 'I see ya, caught ya red-'anded, caught ya red-'anded!'

I'm sure his shrieks were heard in the next street. I always tried to give him a good time.

I popped into the parlour to say my farewells when our game finished. Mr Wing said the usual, 'Sssssshan't keep you, doctor.' He knew I needed to dash off.

Sometime later, Mr Wing died. We expected it, but not so soon. With her Bright's disease, Mrs Black was not able to care for a nephew who was a few sheep short of a flock, so George was hauled off, along with his record player and squeeze box.

I miss playing with Georgie. Mrs Black mentions him whenever I see her.

I got out of the habit of calling in on Mrs Winifred Black after her brother died and her nephew was taken away. She lived alone and preferred it that way. The only surviving blood relative she was permitted to see was the bringer of faith to the grieving Wing teenagers after their parents had been run down. Winifred saw this cousin as little as possible.

One ruse she contrived to continue living independently was to mail herself a postcard every day, requiring Gerard the postman to knock on her door. None of the old houses had letter boxes. One day, no one answered, so Gerard rang me at home. I dashed over, and soon confirmed that the house was shut.

No one answered our pounding, so I popped back home and telephoned. No reply. I returned to the Black house. The postie and I looked at each other, grinned and decided to do some housebreaking. As the slimmer of the two, I climbed in through a hole we made in the front window and unlatched the door. We crept into the silent house, peering into rooms and fearing the worst. Sure enough, Mrs Black was lying on the kitchen floor with a rug wrapped round her and the electric fire blazing nearby. She was in pain from a fractured neck of femur, but quite warm. I cranked her into a comfortable position and, fearing dehydration, put the kettle on. I made time for a cup of tea that day, which the three of us drank on the kitchen floor. Mrs Black told us she left to post the card to herself in the postbox across the road from her gate. When she got home, she took off her coat and shoes and slipped on the stone floor, where she'd been lying for 14 hours.

This episode made her realise that she was not able to live alone. That's when Cousin descended and Mrs Black's downhill slide accelerated in earnest. She was in her 80s, had a good run and now accepted defeat – an all-too-familiar litany I hated to hear.

I resumed visits and postponed wrenching that poor woman from her home. The cousin and her offspring imposed their presence constantly through a sort of twisted compassion that made it impossible to consult with Mrs Black candidly. They were always hovering. She wanted desperately to see her older brother, the university lecturer, one last time.

'What's that in your hand?' I asked one day. I'd purposely come earlier so that the cousin was away at morning ablutions.

Her face lit up. 'Jamie,' she whispered, unfolding her fingers from their treasure. 'But don't let *them* see.' It was the fragment torn from the old photograph in the parlour. 'They won't let me talk to him,' she said. 'Doctor, if it's not too much to ask, could you possibly arrange . . . oh, I shouldn't ask. I have to do as they say. It's what God wants . . . isn't it?'

I was willing to track down Mrs Black's brother, but who was I to come between family members? Where did my duty lie? Other doctors contact excommunicated family members and never doubt their decisions. I couldn't do it.

Winifred Black went to her grave without the comfort of hearing her Jamie's voice one last time. I'd nothing against these folk individually, but it infuriated me that their religion, which espoused to be Christian, was in fact so breathtakingly callous.

Did I do the right thing? I ask myself, and I am not a wondering sort of man.

A lot of water flowing

Amaranth Fillet

Honoured my sister in New York City with a visitation. She married an advertising executive who pulls an amazing salary to entice people to purchase useless goods, or bads. Combined familial duty with a Little Richard concert and a medical conference, where I ran into Tommy MacDonald. We played hookey on our last day. Tommy was mad for indigenous art and I went gaga over the city's architecture, those glittering gems. Precious metals were coaxed from the ground back home, where life was quieter and less public. After 4 days of sirens and the aural detritus of compacted human life 24/7, I yearned for my Antipodean Wild West, that lunar landscape dotted with hermits and others displaced by war and deposited at the ends of the earth, misfits with whom I identified.

Bare lunar hills camouflaged life in those pitted mountains. Inside, miners hacked away, enticing gold, silver, copper, tin, nickel, zinc or lead from the rock face. Caverns sheltered hermits from human contact. People were self-sufficient in the grim way of the monosyllabic needy, without the gentleness of the verbose idealistic.

Diet was a problem. It lacked variety. People preferred fatty foods, and long-distance transport of fresh foods was expensive and hazardous, especially in bad weather. Some people coaxed vegetables out of the rocky soil, but our harsh climate meant a short growing season. Others, like Mick Doherty, found their precious substances and sustenance on top of the ground, in the leavings of their fellow man.

Mick Doherty served in the Second World War and was a bit touched. Those two facts may or may not have been related, depending on who was talking and their mood. When Wayne and I first settled here, Mick lived in a tiny shack on the tip site, where people disposed of their rubbish. He survived on the food scraps he foraged. The town knew his ways and let him live out his days in his chosen fashion, as they wanted to be left alone with their own idiosyncrasies. More than one local threw away perfectly good food, especially in winter, but would have denied it if confronted.

Kids will be kids. They continually annoyed the old man, so Bill Grey, one of the two local grocers, organised a little garden-shed dwelling by the upper reaches of the river that flowed through our town. You crossed several childproof streams to reach Mick's new place. I heard the old veteran was quite happy because he had a chimney.

Late one morning, the grocer rang me at the surgery. 'Can you go out and see Mick Doherty? His legs are swollen up.'

'Long as he doesn't object to being examined by a woman.'

'Didn't think your husband was available.'

'He's not.' This was not the place for feminist heebie-jeebies, and besides, I preferred my humanity to be non-PC. 'Can you give me directions?' I asked. It may have waited until lunch, but the morning was bursting with whingeing tourists and I welcomed a break.

'I'll show you the way. Wear your gumboots.'

Soon we were wading through several streams, each leading deeper into the stubbly mountainside. An image materialised of my sister in her Manhattan apartment, tottering out to off-Broadway shows in her Jimmy Choos. My black rubber boots displaced water like the *Titanic*. I marvelled at the divergence of sororal paths, until a sharp rock projecting like an iceberg demanded my attention. Ferns laced the banks, frozen in various lifelike postures, playing a gigantic game of primeval musical chairs.

Bill Grey – never Bill or Mr Grey, always both names – pulled me and my doctor's bag up the slippery bank into a clearing from which a tin hut poked its chimney, a lush pocket of nature for the old soldier. The grocer was one of the local heroes of our town, to me at least. You'd never pick it from looking at him. I pegged him for Mr Homeless stealing fruit the first time I saw him pawing desiccated oranges and pockmarked apples near the front of his store. He was small and slight, not big and fleshy as you'd expect from someone whose god was food. He wore a battered felt bush hat that hid his eyes and hair. His jacket knew better days 30 years ago. His thick white beard warmed his clavicles and sent the more sensitive townspeople rushing to the other grocer with shudders of hairs in milk and other impossible places. Whether factual or not, it was true in local legend. Another justification for fatty fried foods.

We watched the grey plume from Mr Doherty's little Morsø wood heater twirl and dissipate in the clearing, vanishing in a silver puff. My husband, Wayne, taught me about interstices and not rushing madly forward, so I took a few moments and breathed. The lesson finally took after 15 years of marriage.

'Why are you chuckling, Bill?'

'D'ya know what you're hummin'?'

'"All Australian men need a shed."'

'You're the most musical doc we ever had.'

If only they knew.

Bill Grey frowned as we clumped towards the dwelling. 'Listen, doc.'

'I don't hear anything.'

'That's the point. I don't like it.'

'What do you mean?'

'It's too quiet, doc. Mick usually has his radio on. Hope he's okay.'

We knocked. No answer. Once inside, I looked around. The mattress on the floor must have been cold in the winter. A battered square table lacked a leg and one cane chair had lost half its webbing. They were the only furnishings. Just as well: there wasn't room for anything else, like a kitchen or a stove. Mick boiled his kettle and cooked his food on the cast-iron wood heater with squirrels on the sides. My sister's stark white apartment and red, black and chrome Manhattan galley kitchen tunnelled through my mind.

'Why'd you bring the lady doctor? Where's her husband?' Mr Doherty asked. 'I can talk to him.'

'He's out at the clinic all day, Mick. I checked for you.'

'I'm not taking me clothes off for a woman, not like this.'

'Whatever you want, Mr Doherty. From what Bill Grey said, that won't be necessary.'

'Don't trick me.'

'I won't, Mr Doherty.'

'Nobody calls me that 'cept you and your husband.'

'What shall I call you?'

'Doesn't matter.'

'I was worried, Mick,' the grocer said. 'Didn't hear the radio when we was comin' up.'

The old hermit grunted and scratched his head with clawed fingers bunching up his hair between thumb and fingers.

'Let's sit on the bed, Mr Doherty, so I can examine you.'

'I won't lie down.'

'You don't have to.'

He complied reluctantly, without that combination of alacrity and docility I knew so well. His trousers and shirt emitted the aroma of protective grime that insulates against the cold.

'Let's remove that right boot and sock.' I referred courteously to what passed as footwear.

'That's all?'

'That's all.'

Off they came.

I wriggled and bent his little toe, checking for proprioception, that feeling of joint movement. The long nerves were the most vulnerable and usually went first.

'Can't feel much, doc.'

'This?' I ran a piece of cotton wool over the tops of his toes.'

'Naw.'

'What about this?' I pricked the bottom of his middle toe with a pin.

'Not that neither.'

I suspected glove-and-stocking anaesthesia – neuropathy – that decreased sensation in the hands and feet, so I continued my tests up the leg, looking for the spot at which it suddenly became normal. Mick winced when I pricked his knee. 'Seems a little loose, Mr Doherty. Have you hurt your knee?' I decided not to test for knee-jerk.

'Don't know.'

He dislocated the patella and never fixed it. Must have been painful at the time.

'Your legs are swollen and you have decreased sensation,' I said.

He grunted.

'What do you eat, Mr Doherty?'

'You women are always on about food.'

'I give him leftovers from the grocery shop, mostly tinned stuff,' Bill Grey said. The hermit nodded.

'Do you eat any fresh stuff?' I asked.

Mick shrugged his shoulders. Bill Grey said all in one breath, 'I bring him potatoes and cabbage and sometimes onions and oranges and whatever else is around but I've found them dumped outside here so the answer to your question is no.'

'Give him some vitamin B₁ tablets and see if he'll eat fresh fruit and vegetables.' The hermit might be thiamine-deficient, so I took some blood.

As we were going, the grocer asked, 'Where's that radio I gave you for company, Mick?'

He mumbled something.

The grocer leaned forward. 'What was that, mate?'

'I drowned it.'

'What?'

'I chucked it in the water and watched it sink. Real satisfyin' it was.'

'Why'd you do that?'

'It was that woman.'

'What woman?'

'The one on the wireless. She was annoying me.'

'But you like listening to the radio.'

'Not her. She didn't belong out here. She grated.'

At the time, Pru Beckley hosted a talkback radio show. She'd a notably abrasive voice.

'So you drowned your radio because you loathed her voice,' I said.

He nodded. I appreciated his control over his aural environment, so unlike my sister's.

'Be sure and tell your husband you saw me. I want his opinion.'

Mick's results came back and sure enough it was beriberi. That afflicted prisoners at Changi in the Second World War and mainly hermits and alcoholics in the West nowadays. Hubby Wayne took out some vitamins and fresh vegetables, with instructions that Bill Grey was to watch Mr Doherty consume them and report back. To my knowledge, nary another radio crossed the old hermit's path. Sure enough, he got better. His legs eventually returned to normal.

Mr Doherty eventually ended up in town. Being out on the river was a younger man's game. He was quite happy to be in an abandoned house near the hospital, with a roof and floor and a fireplace and a few walls, but no electricity or running water.

One day, some official objected to his living conditions, so we put him into our nursing home at the hospital. Before long, he caused an incident with a television that annoyed the staff. The superintendent kicked him out. The newspaper ran a story on the hard-hearted bureaucrat who had turfed out this nice old guy. Mick quite happily returned to his abandoned house. I used to go out to check if he'd hurt or injured himself.

A year later a nurse rang from a nearby town. 'We've got this guy down here, lives with his brother, they're both hermits, and he's got swollen legs and he may not be able to feel them.' I said, 'Thiamine deficiency.' She said, 'What?!' I said, 'I reckon he's got beriberi.' 'How can you say that over the telephone?' 'I bet I'm right.' So I went over and took his blood, and it was thiamine deficiency.

The nurse was flabbergasted. 'Give me a hard one to solve next time!' I said. I've never seen beriberi again.

Wayne and I shared other patients whose lives were contorted by the Second World War, like the Wallinskys. In them unravelled our future, the end of the line of the mass delusion called *And they lived happily ever after.*

'I hate you!' Mrs Wallinsky shrieked. If looks could kill. 'I want revenge.' She was a large woman, placid until her mind started to go, and robust in that sensible European way that included massages and the tisanes cherished by Hercule Poirot.

'She's not herself, doctor,' Mr Wallinsky said in a small, wounded voice. What he meant was that he'd reached his limit. The poor man was developing his own problems as he aged – they were in their 70s – and, like his wife's, they weren't all physical.

We were sitting round the kitchen table over a cup of tea and home-made goodies. Some months before, I'd started popping round. I didn't want to add to Mr W's burden by making him dress her properly and bring her to the surgery. I enjoyed going out. The window over the sink framed the river that defined our town. At that time, Mick Doherty still lived rough a few bends and twists away. Mrs Wallinsky treasured this view, the best in the house, she claimed. Little pleasures and triumphs comprised a happy life.

The traditional number of afternoon-tea offerings adorned the table: two kinds of home-made biscuits, oatmeal (stale) and ginger (burnt), fruit cake (over-cooked) – one of those Brit concoctions that can be thrown at the wall without breaking – ham sandwiches (dry) and courgette loaf (soggy in the middle). All stood in mute salute to the declining powers of the woman of the house.

Missing from the table were *oliebollen* from the old country, which Mrs Wallinsky no longer made. Their absence changed the aromas in her kitchen. No more bubbling oil in the frying pan transforming little balls of batter into hot doughnuts piled high on a plate and dusted with icing sugar. As Mrs W relinquished her grip on our shared reality, her table began to smell of Desiccating Empire Outpost, with offerings hundreds of years old. The oil-and-sugar combinations of European and British life were ripped from her competence on the journey to a different land. That it was terrifying and lonely shone from her eyes. Mrs W's afternoon tea evoked different fragrances from those of Mrs Eastley, the vicar's wife in Sussex, which were unlike those permeating the patisseries of New York City and the backwaters of the Caribbean. As for the islands where I did a locum for Petra Neumann, all I can recall is the underlying, overarching stench of mutton fat in apple-tart pastry and sultana cake, which took some habituating to and which no amount of cream could disguise.

That day, Mr Wallinsky was ground into weary submission. 'It's the same old argument, dear. Please come to terms with this.'

'Don't give me an ultimatum.' Sez she. Don't blame her.

'I'm too drained at the end of the day for this.' Poor guy.

Turn to the doctor.

'He's always out in his bloody shed anyway.'

'She refuses to acknowledge that she's losing it.'

Turn back to each other.

'You idiot! I am not!'

'See what I mean? Yesterday she was reading her women's magazine upside down.'

'I was only spacing out! Everyone does that.'

'For 2 hours?'

'It wasn't that long. It was only a few minutes.'

'I checked the kitchen clock on my way to the shed. You were in the same place when I came back in at morning-tea time.'

'So what? What are you, the activity police?'

'I'm worried about you.'

'Leave me alone. Stop hectoring me.'

'I'm your husband. I love you.'

'Stop acting like a gaoler.'

Each knotted face mirrored the other's pain. We all looked out the window at the river view, composing ourselves for the next round in the inexorable war we were all destined to lose. How to explain the eroding inhibition of senile dementia, *the losses*, piling up day by day by day? This was not the moment to mention the Alzheimer's disease that claimed Mrs Wallinsky's mother. *Remember to remove 'Where've You Been?' from the iPod, girl. Can't stand Kathy Mattea chirruping about a devoted couple now living on different hospital floors after 60 years without a night apart. Sob.*

Mr Wallinsky sloshed down his teacup and stormed out, calling back, 'I'll be in the shed.' Years of emotional yo-yoing might snap anyone's elastic patience or dissolve the social glue that pinioned certain fleeting feelings in the dark.

I examined a photograph of a broad-faced ruddy young man in a wedding scene in the one photograph that survived the Second World War and dislocation to an alien culture. That silver-plated image took pride of place on the window ledge over the sink, where she could see him when she washed up. His blonde, northern European looks were attractive in youth but faded quickly. His eyes paled to a lustreless blue. The high cheekbones remained and gave his face an exotic dignity in old age. Next to him a young girl gazed up adoringly. She wore a brooch which looked like a family treasure, an ornament she wore every time we met outside the home, at fêtes, functions and in the surgery.

I've a time of it to recall when she last came in to see me, never during flu season for a needle, as the locals called it. The Wallinskys were childless, so experienced no kiddie broken arms, sprained ankles or disabilities, mental or physical. Her devastating illness turned her husband desperate. She affixed the brooch sideways or upside down – she, the precise one. Poor Mr Wallinsky once told me that he'd found that treasure in the refrigerator.

'Those oatmeal biscuits look like your *oliebollen*,' I said. 'They were something special.'

The good woman's eyes lit up. 'My grandmother made them 100 years ago.' She frowned. 'Or was it my mother? Or my great-grandmother?'

'You once told me you hid during the war.'

She nodded. 'For a year. My grandfather was a railroad executive, so nobody questioned him much. The Nazis wanted to conscript me. They'd plenty of uses for a 15-year-old girl. But my grandfather wouldn't allow that to happen. Finally, I ran away, and that's how I met' – gesture at the shed – 'himself.' Her eyes circled the table. 'This is so much abundance, after eating tulip bulbs.'

'The Hunger Winter.'

'Yes. He's been protecting me as long as I've known him. But now . . .'

'You're on your own,' I said gently.

She looked down and swallowed.

God how I hate this affliction.

We busied ourselves with the mechanics of pouring and stirring. Rituals provide breathing space and equilibrium and allow patients to retain their dignity.

'I constructed a lifetime of memories to nourish my old age, but most of them torment me now,' she whispered. 'I did so much wrong, which I can never correct. And doctor . . .'

'Yes,' I said, putting my hand on hers.

She looked up at me furtively, quickly, as if ashamed of her words. 'I'm so frightened.'

Mr Wallinsky finally put her into a complete-care facility. She lives on, healthy as ever in body, mind completely gone, and no longer recognises anyone, including her husband.

Last time I saw Mr Wallinsky, he was living alone in the home they had shared for over 40 years. We'd got the health formalities like his glucometer readings out of the way and were lingering over a cup of tea at the kitchen table, where he now spent most of his days. This was his wife's territory, and her ghost dominated the room. Gone was the scrubbed tabletop laden with fragrant pastry dough, marble rolling pins and bowls of filling and glaze. Newspapers, books and half-filled notepads now claimed it, along with forgotten cups of tea. He was adrift in the way of those elderly who have lost a spouse and feel a phantom limb after major amputation. Rotating his situation in a certain light made my eyes tear over. *Stop it, girl. Jump off the road to temptation and pain. Banish Mrs Eastley in Sussex from your consciousness. CBT – cognitive behavioural therapy – think of your kiddies. You're useless to your patient this way.* I scoured my brain for a Little Richard song to distract me but found none.

The rain pelted down all day. Through the window over the sink, we watched the river jump.

'You know, doctor,' Mr W said, 'the Vedas regard water, present in air, rain, mist and clouds, as the tangible manifestation of the divine presence.' The poor man was thirsting for conversation. 'Have you read any of Masaru Emoto's research?'

'Didn't he photograph frozen water and write accompanying meditations, Mr Wallinsky?' I'd never call him Stanislav or Stan, as he was known, or his wife Anselina or Lina. Some patients liked formality with their doctors.

'Sort of. He photographed water crystals at the moment of freezing and showed the direct consequences of destructive and loving thoughts on the crystals' formation.'[8]

'I remember hearing that a water crystal forms and disappears in 120 seconds.'

'Emoto and his team showed words to a beaker of water. Words and phrases like Hate, Happiness, Love, You Idiot! and Thank You in various languages were reflected in the water. Startlingly different crystal formed. They used city water, dam water and dew from a piece of bamboo on a mountain trail. Water

8 Emoto 2005.

not allowed to flow dies. A crystal formed from pond water from a planned land-reclamation area looks tortured and miserable.'

'So what does it all mean, Mr Wallinsky?'

'You're the one with the answers, Dr Fillet, you tell me.'

'Not by a long shot, Mr Wallinsky, not I.'

'Tell me why I can't protect my wife anymore.' He turned away, but not before I saw major desolation and abandonment in his eyes. 'It's all a man wants,' he said, voice cracking. He gazed out at the river. Best view in the house. 'I played the game like I was supposed to and now look.'

'I'd give anything to wave a magic wand to make it all disappear, Mr Wallinsky. The time for words is past. Stroke her hair and let whatever good you can ripple through your fingers.'

'I've seen a lot of water flow under a lot of bridges and I still haven't found the source.'

I headed home for comfort. I logged on to the Internet and clicked my most used bookmark. Before long some loved words soothed me from cyberspace: 'Hi, this is Little Richard. I want to say hello to all of my fans all over the world. I love you so much . . .'

Mr Wallinsky

Wayne Cooperville

'Sorry I'm late,' Wayne Cooperville said. 'Ah, you've ordered your food already. I've been shopping. My daughter wants some sort of American Indian object with copious pink feathers. Now, I ask you. And she needs, absolutely has to have a statue of a dancing Shiva for her altar. *My* daughter. I understand adolescent rebellion, but have I failed so completely to instil in her a love of reason? She gets it from her mother, along with that sense of otherness. My first wife was so grounded.'

'Mr Wallinsky, it's me, Dr Cooperville,' I called into the house by the river late one spring day. The weather was freakish for the time of year, with hideous winds and rogue frosts withering tomato seedlings lovingly coaxed into life across the north of the state.

I'm not often out this way, but I decided to call in on Mr Wallinsky on the way home from a visit to a sick child. Truth be told, I wanted to postpone going home. Amaranth was planning to work in Mrs Eastley's Sussex village. A letter from the old lady arrived the previous day. An early-morning phone call informed me that a massive stroke claimed the vicar's wife and could I please inform Dr Amaranth Fillet at the specific request of the deceased? I dreaded it. She'd blame me. It's true, I was partly responsible, forcing her to choose between me and the children and that sweet old woman to whom she'd given a pledge. Please God, don't let this send my wife off the deep end, back into the world of drugs. I'd put in an urgent call to her Uncle Zoltan and was now hoping for a message at the surgery or at home.

Such were my jumbled recriminations and prayers as I strode up the walk of a lonely old man with a wife beyond his reach, despite the desperate wishes of them both.

A knock on the door sent him running for his shotgun – either that or into hiding. I became astute at judging whether his footfall was terrified or violent. Frantic, scurrying footsteps told me that Mr Wallinsky's paranoia was worsening as he got older. It was hideous for everyone when our patients contracted such modern scourges as Alzheimer's disease. Combine that heartbreak with the life of an immigrant who never fit in, and whose wife we'd put into a home the year before. She no longer recognised her saviour from the Second World War. They had only each other for all those years, and now not even that. Now, she stared out of a window that didn't open at a fountain that was turned off at 5 p.m. each day. He stared out of her kitchen window, alone, alone.

Immigrants bring us treasures from their cultures, if only we're open to them. Their approach to health and medicine can be radically different. Some of my colleagues react with contempt, amusement, condescension and anger to alternative medicine. 'Patients come to us when they're really sick,' they say, 'and sometimes they've delayed it too long with that quackery.' My dear wife Amaranth can be quite scathing about my lack of acceptance of alternative medicine, but everything's all right in its place.

I caught the tail end of the displaced-person influx from Hungary, Czechoslovakia and the Baltic states. Amaranth's Uncle Zoltan told us about Kazimiera Aspakich from Lithuania, who'd survived the Russian Revolution and the invasion of his country by the Russians, followed by the Germans and then the Russians again. He'd escaped from Lithuania and eventually come to the middle of Europe in winter in 1945, and ended up here as a displaced person.

I can hear Zoltan as if he were here, and can do no better than to give him the floor: 'This gent did well here, and was the proud owner of a lovely house with beautiful things. I'm not a great "beautiful things" man. One picture is much the same as the next one, but I recognised that his pictures were masterfully painted and his cabinet work was exquisite. I suppose word got out. One day, a gentleman arrived with a shotgun and a couple of mates to raid the house. What they didn't know was that my old patient was a survivor. They grabbed his wife and hit her with a gun. To frighten him was the idea. So, he played the craven middle European, wringing his hands, "Oh, don't hurt us, ve be all right, I go for de money straight away." He crept off. They foolishly stayed put. Unfortunately for them, he came back with a .45 revolver and blew a hole in them! Stone dead.' Uncle Zoltan extended his forefinger and cocked his thumb. 'Boing! Being well into his 80s, they deemed him too old to plead in court and fined him for possessing an unlicensed firearm. It doesn't pay to tackle ancient gentlemen who may be fitter than you think! And certainly not to hit their wives.'

These displaced families were often social isolates, with a husband and wife but no family, like Mr and Mrs Wallinsky. Now the old man was alone, with the numb bewilderment of the elderly bereaved I'd observed so often in the surviving spouse. In my experience, men tend to be more dependent.

A flutter in the sitting room to the right of the door caught my eye as I knocked that spring day. I did something of which I'm ashamed, which catapulted me into the interstices between two worlds and left me incapable of propelling myself forward or backward. It left me petrifying in the Biblical sense. I threaded through the shrubs, peered inside and stood rooted to the spot. Having my privacy disrupted drives me demented, so why was I intruding upon a patient's? I was disregarding a marker of civilisation, something of which I'd righteously accused wife Amaranth and the children on numerous occasions when they overran my shed (actually, my office out the back, which began life as the garden shed that Mr Wallinsky left me in his will). Here I was, doing the same to a patient, and a paranoid one at that. No one likes being surprised in a private moment. A mini-revenge was telling the neighbours: 'My doctor was spying on me.'

A vision riveted me into place, driving another bolt into the doctor–patient relationship. It was nothing dramatic. A public defender would have found nothing criminal in an elderly man shuffling towards a cold, dark fireplace. A journalist may have yawned at the sight of hands burrowed deep in cardigan pockets, shoulders hunched, eyes down.

I, however, was trained differently, and I didn't like what I saw. My patient stood before the chipped mantel, deep in animated conversation with a photograph of his wife on their wedding day. In happier times, it perched between the sink and the window in the kitchen. This object which symbolised happiness for so long became a bittersweet survivor, like the human supplicant before it. The large stain on the back of his cardigan was not a good sign. His wife wouldn't have tolerated such a thing.

Mr Wallinsky never visited his wife. She didn't recognise him. It was too painful. He could no longer protect the only person he loved. I thought about Amaranth and the children and swallowed the lump in my throat.

The crashings of the rubbish-collection truck broke the spell cementing us in place. Mr Wallinsky glanced up and busted me.

'Mr Wallinsky,' I said, embarrassed. Best not to justify my action, but to ignore it. My upbringing taught me that. Amaranth scolded that I should stop blaming my parents. 'I'll go to the door here.'

Mr Wallinsky had solidified into a wizened little man with a certain neatness exemplified by a perfectly trimmed grey moustache. He always wore a hat over his balding head and carried a walking stick.

He taught me something about pride. Both he and his wife were extremely house-proud in the days before the disease of time ensnared them.

Soon the front door opened a crack, revealing the butt of a shotgun and my patient's eyes.

'I'm alone,' I said. 'Your name was on the patient list for this afternoon. I'm out this way and wanted to save you a trip.'

'It's warm in the kitchen.' He spoke in heavily accented English and gestured me inside.

'Okay.'

I followed his shuffling form down the hall. We entered the kitchen in the back of the house. He gestured me to a battered wooden table. I sat, putting my medical bag next to me.

He pulled out a chair across from me. He chose to overlook my bad behaviour and commented instead on my attire. Patients notice when a shirt is ironed. 'You've lifted your game, doctor. Usually, your clothes are wrinkled.'

'Amaranth doesn't iron, I'm afraid.' It was one of the chores of Mrs Clarke, who *does* for us, but her priorities were cleaning up after two adults and four children. I contrasted myself with Mr Wallinsky, whose wife had always kept him neat and dapper: easier for him, with his slight build, than for my stocky and bearish body. That my shirts floated on a layer of body hair mesmerised children and fascinated my wife. I'd found it difficult to be 5 feet 8 inches tall and a little shorter than Amaranth in a culture in which height mattered, but Amaranth didn't care. She insisted that we'd shrink together blissfully into old age.

'I hear you've sold the house,' I said.

'That's right, doctor,' he said. 'Built it myself over 40 years ago, so I know it's solid.' His 25 years with the Forestry Commission made him a deft hand with a chainsaw. He was one of those fortunate people who excelled at whatever they tried.

'I'm not sad I sold it. The missus and I spent 43 years here full of wonderful memories. The last two were so bad I am glad to leave. Thank you for getting her into Restful Haven.'

He was right. The house was nothing like in Mrs Wallinsky's reign. No cooking aromas or tang of floor wax, no bustling activity or scolding for tracking in dirt. Now no one visited Mr Wallinsky, and he returned the favour.

'Thank you for coming, doctor,' he said, voice rusty and strained from disuse.

'No worries, Mr Wallinsky.' I leaned down to open my black bag.

He searched in a dresser drawer. 'Here are some chocolates for your little ones.' He always found something for our children.

'Four daughters,' he chuckled.

'Four little Amaranths, God help me.'

The old man placed the sweets on the table and extracted some paper. 'My charts, doctor.' He set his diabetic records neatly in front of me. He kept them obsessively.

I flipped through the pages.

'You've been measuring your urine twice a day,' I said approvingly. He'd have measured it 10 times a day if we asked him.

'Yes, doctor, that glucometer makes all the difference.' We'd got him one a few months before and he loved it.

We discussed depression, but he rejected it in any form. 'Are you sleeping okay, Mr Wallinsky?'

'As well as can be expected under the circumstances, doctor.'

'How's your appetite?'

'How do you think, now that I have to cook for myself?'

'Perhaps we should pop you into hospital for a few days for a good going-over.'

His snort took us back to the haunting interstices.

I'd learned over the years that sometimes it was best to let patients be. 'Do you need anything, Mr Wallinsky?' I asked.

'No, Fred looks after me and the boys chop my wood. I'm quite content.'

Fred, our ambulance officer, made Mr Wallinsky's last years his most tranquil since coming to this country. Fred is a bloody saint. Every night, he tucked Mr Wallinsky into bed. Because Mr Wallinsky was different, kids knocked at his door and ran away. He started coming to the door with a knife or any weapon at hand.

'The boys?'

'They're okay now, doctor.'

Fred realised that all the boys wanted was to see the old fellow, so he set them to chopping Mr Wallinsky's wood.

'Remember the shed, doctor. I won't finalise the sale of this place until then.'

That shed was the sole footprint of his time on earth. I once knew a lady who was obsessed with an ancient double sink. She willed it to her nurse, who refused to haul it away when the old woman was alive. After she died, her nephews sold it to those human scavengers who plague the homes of the recently dead – as the old lady had feared.

'I won't, Mr Wallinsky,' I said softly. 'I'm on call this weekend, there's a conference the next one and I promised to take Amaranth and the children away after that – I simply *must* – but are you available at the end of the month?'

'Whatever suits you, doctor. I've got all the time in the world.'

This wasn't strictly true. Mr Wallinsky died on our family weekend away. I didn't expect it quite so soon, but I knew he was ready.

The shed was designed quite differently from the ones in this country, and was painted that light blue favoured by some Europeans. As I was clearing it out in preparation for its move, I found two paintings. The first was a beauty. I nearly missed it, as he'd wrapped in an old sheet and stuck it in a corner. Dust rose as I lifted the sheet and gazed at Mrs Wallinsky in her hearty prime, brooch pinned precisely over her left breast. She smiled at the painter through the steam generated by apricots stewing on the stove, which she stirred with a wooden spoon gripped in her competent hand. I knew of no one to inherit the painting, which is just as well, because Amaranth snatched it up and hung it in her office, next to her diplomas and a map of world music.

The second painting stopped me in my tracks: an unfinished oil of the three boys who first harassed Mr Wallinsky and subsequently chopped his wood. It captured perfectly the mischief and energy of boyhood. A blonde boy clutched a rock in his right fist, poised to throw. His dark-haired mate wielded an axe over a block of wood. The third looked into the distance, hands unfinished.

I hung the painting in my new blue shed, over my desk, where I look at it whenever I lean back. Unlike my wife, I did not place it on view for my patients. Some conversations are private.

Whitefella dreaming 3 ━━━

Tommy MacDonald

Violence against doctors is on the rise, with murders making the news. In the United States, it's the terminators; in Australia, three GPs have been murdered in the last decade. One was a female Druze with a devastated young family; the second a male doing a home visit; the third a European immigrant who fatally stabbed his partner and lived on after a botched murder-suicide attempt. A paranoid schizophrenic patient terrorised Petra Neumann. I faced Young Edward.

But for Eddie Mayfield, I'd be another statistic. Perhaps I am anyway. I'd been working 3 weeks on, 3 weeks off for years in the desert east of Western Australia, without encountering any violence directed against myself, until Young Edward sniffed petrol one too many times.

Back inside my painting. Old Faye and Young Faye were in the waiting room with her toddler. A video player spun out a health-education lesson at top volume, because people tended to be hard of hearing and there was a lot of noise. Eddie sat in the consulting room with his mouth around a spirometer.

'You know what to do,' I said, clipping a peg on his nose.

'I won't let any air out through my mouth.' The old man adjusted his lips round the mouthpiece.

'I'll count to three, and I want you to blow out hard, get all the air out of your lungs and inhale as much as you can, holding it to the count of 10.'

With a little ingenuity, I had obtained a spirometer for testing lung function. People loved their motorcars out here and spent a lot of money on them. It was a harsh environment for vehicles – rough roads, dusty – and they broke down sooner rather than later. Each community made room for a graveyard of dead motorcars. A lot of their wheels were magnesium alloy, so I recycled metal for a couple of years, along with radiators and bull bars. One day, I backloaded a store-supply truck – which returned empty to Perth, 2000 kilometres away – and sold it all at one of the scrap-metal yards. I raised $2500. With that, we bought two spirometers, one for the eastern group of communities and one for the western. Tommy McD's little metal-recycling business! I filled up the Toyota with bloody radiators and mag wheels I collected, and bought a roof rack from an Aboriginal in another community, for aluminium bull bars.

'Blow, Eddie, blow, blow, out, out, out and in, *in* and hold it one, two, three . . .'

Reduced lung functions due to chronic infections, smoking, petrol sniffing and inhalation of smoke from campfires – or a combination of the above – was not unusual. There's no tuberculosis. That's more Top End, with leprosy, where there's an animal reservoir in pigs and buffalos and such. Someone with a chronic disease has to have a contextual grasp of what it means for his future, or he's going to have trouble understanding why he needs to take medication regularly, not only for 1 week but perhaps for the next 17 years. That's another example of people in this transitional period between their world view and ours.

'Keep holding Eddie, holding, holding, six, seven . . .'

World-view issues surface regularly. It's difficult to ask a white woman if her husband's been beating her, or innocuous questions like, 'Are you still smoking cigarettes?' or 'How often do you feel the pain?' It's challenging when people's numerical context is different to ours, not to mention a dissimilar concept of time and their understanding of relationships and consequent strengths and value. It becomes arduous when many people have chronic disease, like out here: cardiovascular, kidney and lung as well as diabetes, illnesses which are not going to improve.

'Almost there, nine, 10 and blow, blow, blow, get it all out, keep going, and going, and stop. Breathe normally while I set up the last test.'

Eddie pushed the breathing apparatus away and sat back with a satisfied thump. One ordeal was over. He watched me impassively as I prepared for the next.

Hang on. Back up.

Something was wrong.

I shouldn't have heard that gentle movement of Eddie's. The waiting room was too quiet.

The front door of the clinic banged open. An aggressive young male voice dominated a crash of glass and metal. The video player stopped. It was Young Edward.

I froze, turning my eyes without moving my head to look at Eddie, who was looking down. 'Petrol sniffer,' he mumbled.

I looked out the window, hoping that the policeman was on his rounds. Instead I saw a discarded petrol tin upended in the road. I'd been so absorbed in Eddie's lung function tests I'd not noticed a kerfuffle in the street. I wished for a guard dog or capsicum spray, like some of my colleagues used on out-of-hours callouts and hospital or surgery visits. 'Like his brothers,' Eddie said. One of Young Edward's elder brothers was in a permanent vegetative state in a nursing home in Alice Springs, his brain melted from sniffing leaded petrol. He was otherwise healthy and could expect to live for many years, at a cost to the taxpayer of $160 000 per year. I heard of a demonstration of the effects of petrol sniffing on the fatty tissue of the brain. Someone poured petrol over a saucer of butter, which it rapidly melted.

The same addiction caused the death of another brother, to whom Young Edward was closest, while the teenager was in prison 500 kilometres away for grievous bodily harm. He turned nasty under the influence and attacked someone with a star picket, the closest thing to hand, because they wouldn't let him return to bury his brother. Now he was grieving and 'chroming.' His mother was out drinking somewhere. Young Edward's home life was full of sorry business, violence and poverty. Combined with boredom and petrol's availability and affordability, small wonder he started sniffing petrol socially at the age of seven with his older brothers, who cared for him while their mother was out cold on the sofa.

I heard Old Faye and Young Faye in the waiting room with her toddler. Eddie and I rushed to the consulting room door as Young Faye ran through the front one, clutching her baby. Old Faye slid along the wall to follow.

'Edward,' I said to distract him. He looked at me. I gestured for Old Faye to run for it.

He clutched a crowbar as he turned to face me. 'Try to escape, Eddie!' I hissed from the side of my mouth.

'No,' came the firm reply.

The woman made it to freedom. I was on my own. I might be able to get some diazepam down Young Edward, but I doubted it.

'The police were watching me through that' – he gestured at the shattered video – 'and now they're coming out of your hair!' He raised the crowbar.

'Edward,' I said, putting my arms out slowly, 'why don't you give me that before you hurt yourself? Let's talk.'

'You can't fool me!' He advanced, all 110 kilogrammes and 6 feet 2 inches of him. He was stripped to the waist, which people often do to show their displeasure. Men and women both. All ages. It's part of the posturing of making your position known.

Eddie was next to me the whole time. He started speaking soothingly, incomprehensibly, in their tongue.

Young Edward registered Eddie's words ever so slightly, hesitated and continued forward. I was a hair's breadth away from being whacked across the face with a crowbar, but he tripped on a blue plastic toy elephant. Going down stunned him long enough for Eddie to crouch down and work his soothing magic. We heaved Young Edward on the examining table and sedated him.

'Gotta build that centre,' Eddie said.

Plans were underway to construct a combined youth, sport and recreational club that provided structured activities to engage young people, enhance their self-esteem, promote indigenous culture and develop a sense of community. Or so they said.

'And a healing place,' Eddie continued. 'Otherwise there'll be no young people to carry on when we go.'

The government was addressing the problem of petrol sniffing among the young. First, it tackled the community's drinking problems to enable affected parents to provide care and guidance to their offspring. We needed culturally appropriate places for abusers which gave them time to heal, like the Maori healing ones in New Zealand. There was one place for young people a few hundred kilometres northwest of Alice Springs, far from abuse substances, for rehab and detox under the supervision of their elders. I think they were taught droving skills. Communities that worked with cattle experienced fewer problems with substance abuse. Animals were healing, and gave them something to stave off boredom, and a pay cheque and structure and self-esteem. Participating in work, recreation and leisure programmes far from home was supposed to address the young people's physical, spiritual and social needs. That it was based on a cultural model of banishment made it appropriate.

I needed time away. I was thankful to be doing remote clinics the next day. A night under the stars would restore my equilibrium. I shouldn't have driven the troop carrier, as I felt anxious and my concentration was poor. Easy to say, using Zoltan Nagy's retrospectoscope. Flashbacks crept into my consultations for the rest of the day. My judgement was affected.

I'll go back as soon as I can.

Pursued ▬▬▬

Dexter Veriform

A shadow crossed Dexter Veriform's prison hospital bed and dimmed the shaft of sun from barred window. 'The guardian of righteousness,' he grunted. 'Light and dark, right and wrong. Doctors and police have a lot in common. We authority figures are called out at all hours for people's life crises. This extracts a toll on our families; both professions have high divorce rates. We must be obeyed at work, but try that at home and the consequences are unmentionable. And drugs are always close. It's merely a difference of approach.'

I absolutely refuse to let *anyone* intrude upon the doctor–patient relationship, not family, not femocrats, no one. That's sacred. Notice I call them *patients*, not *clients*. That little spasm of rebellion cost me dearly – everything, in fact, as I've said.

After all these years, all those patients, all that work, here I am crossing paths with policedom in an unexpected way which may be the end of me. And again it's drugs, drugs, drugs. Why *wouldn't* I go my own way? Why on earth – hell's bells on airth, as Wee Donnie McKay said back in Scotland – would I allow a bureaucrat with very few years of training under its belt to dictate how I treat my patients? That's why I've ended up in this prison hospital bed. This one happened to be female. Give a little power to somebody with a chip on her shoulder and potentially average intelligence and what happens? They always win in the end, don't they, like cockroaches. I'm a cautionary tale.

It started at a conference I wasn't keen to attend, but I needed the continuing-education points to maintain my medical standing (ahem). Miss Brianna Bugden was the name on her tag. The way she crossed her arms bespoke the humourless, rights-orientated female our *zeitgeist* disgorged. I'd no experience dealing with this new woman. What's the point of feminism? We're all in this together and should contribute in whatever ways we can. Why deflect energy from the mutual slog? So society's rulers can continue to divide and conquer. Keep people at war with one another so they cannot unite against the *real* enemy.

Ms Brianna Bugden's blonde, peroxided spikes and prickly personality accompanied a body as broad as it was long and solid as they come, more a mountain of Parmesan than a mound of Brie. She heard me – *overheard* me – consulting with a colleague about a patient. They lurk at the edges of private conversations, waiting to pounce. I'd looked forward to my colleague's advice as the bright spot in a boring conference.

'Clients!' she roared.

He and I were propelled, dazed, from the depths of our compassion. 'Whatever do you mean?' I asked.

'They're not called patients!' said she, chins aquiver with righteous indignation.

'Madam, you are intruding upon a confidential consultation,' said my esteemed colleague.

'I'll call them whatever I please,' I said, turning my back on this interfering female.

'I know you,' she said.

'Bugden . . . I don't recall . . .' I said, rotating to face this personage.

'My mother was pregnant with me when we left the west coast of Scotland. Daddy brought us out on assisted passage during the White Australia policy.'

No bells rung. 'I'm afraid, as we met when you were in the womb . . .'

'You always called my father *Mister* Whoople. He said you was having him on. He wanted to be called Brian. He showed you that by calling you Dexter.'

The mist parted. Oh, no. Please God, no. Yes. She didn't resemble her father at all, but had inherited the widely set piscine eyes of the two sisters who adored Whoople for some reason.

'He hated you.'

I bit my lip. Better not say that the feeling was mutual.

'And now I've tracked you down,' she said triumphantly. 'I promised Daddy I would, no matter how long it took. My parents heard how you killed that little boy in Scotland.'

My heart froze. Sandy MacSalter's severe disabilities enslaved his little brothers and sisters, not to mention his parents. Meningitis appeared like a ministering angel. I chose to let nature run its course.

'I may not be able to get you for that, but I'll make sure your murderous career ends with Dr X. My only regret is that Daddy is not alive to share in the victory.'

'And your father?' I asked.

'Diabetes took him 4 years ago,' she said, and paused, expecting condolences. I forbore.

'We sued his GP,' she continued, 'because we weren't given enough lifestyle information – a nice little sum we got from the insurance company – and I always promised Daddy I'd get you. Now I've found you, at last. I know about Dr X, and believe me, you're going to pay.'

The importance of the consultation with my colleague diminished into nothingness. 'I don't know what you mean.'

'Oh, yes you do. You killed Dr X. I read the statutory declaration of his son.' Andrew had hated his father and was mentally disturbed. 'It's enough for me to use. We're preparing the case now. I probably shouldn't have brought it up, but I want you to suffer like Daddy.'

That was the beginning of the end and the start of a new sort of doctor–police interaction in my life. Had I known what I know now, would I have lived my life differently? Could I have prevented the mistakes arising from my particular conglomeration of traits, or was I doomed to repeat them over and over? I'll leave eternal recurrence to the philosophers and such other chroniclers of the human condition as PD Ouspensky[9] and Honoré de Balzac.[10]

I've plenty of time to think in here, being locked away as I am. And for what? Doing what a patient wanted and I knew to be right. I've always done what I could when patients beg for help at the end. Usually, it's extra morphine, but not always.

No, not always, as with Dr X. He and I made a pact early on, which I respected. It was one of the ethical dilemmas I faced daily. My decision grew out of the doctor–patient relationship. I even discussed it with Thucydides Hare, who agreed with me. Dr X's terminal disease was not as simple as Mr Stevens' carcinoma of the bowel. I persuaded the latter to kill himself in the open if he insisted on doing it, where it was easier to tidy up the many bits and pieces. Mr Stevens considerately shot himself by the incinerator.

In those days, suicide carried an even bigger stigma. My last ministration to Dr X was to write on his post-mortem report that he'd died of complications from the disease, which was certainly true. That didn't satisfy our femocrat. Mr Whoople's child was determined to prove that I'd euthanised my poor colleague. Who appointed her as watchdog? Do we really want such people as guardians of our morality?

Here's what happened. What would you have done? Do any of us know until thrust into the same situation, as either doctor or patient? We think we know, but just wait.

I called in at Dr X's on my way to the surgery one morning, as I'd got into the habit of doing. I parked facing the orchard, his pride and joy in healthier times, before he contracted multiple sclerosis. Dr X ran and ran and ran, round and round and round, the orchard's worn dirt track, sometimes in the morning before work, sometimes afterwards in the dark.

Dr X was my mentor, generously intertwining my professional life with his. That dreadful disease, much commoner in the higher latitudes, might have lain its gruesome claw on any of us. Dr X's end was very, very sad, for everybody. He'd no self-respect left. He was incontinent. His wife was very willing indeed to look after him, but whatever lay beyond the rainbow bridge beckoned him from the horrific chains indenturing him to this side.

I knew what I'd find today: a 57-year-old general practitioner slightly farther along the downhill track of no return. I hated this part of my work.

His wife showed me in. Mrs X was frayed round the edges, as we all were from this awful disease that had struck our colleague and loved one. Genevieve was a nurse before she married and now tended her husband superbly.

'How are the children coping?' I asked, hoping for the impossible.

'The same,' came the wifely quaver as she tucked the wandering goose-down quilt back under his chin, to keep out the autumn cold. 'Josie barely, Andrew not at all.'

Dr X's daughter would be okay in time. She exemplified the best of doctors' families: the resilience, the empathy and the loyalty. Or am I idealising? Andrew,

9 Ouspensky 1973.
10 Balzac 1963.

on the other hand, did not grow into his considerable potential, drifting from one unskilled job to another. Dr X couldn't discuss his son without a blink of guilt. When we'd initially conferred about the disease's inevitable progress, Dr X whispered his worst regret: that he wouldn't live to see the fullness of time sort out their relationship. As often happens.

'Rrrr.' Dr X's vain efforts to enunciate were painful to behold. He scowled at my doctor's bag.

'You're going through them,' I said gently at his bedside, holding his arm in my two hands. I knew what was going on. Not everything went into my notes.

Dr X lurched through a nightmare from which he expected the worst possible outcome. Its awful grip immobilised him completely, but his mental processes were sharp as ever.

'Rrrr!' Dr X growled fiercely. It was the only means of communication left to a previously articulate man, one who loved the written and spoken word.

I knew what he wanted.

I find this extremely difficult to recall. I'm forcing myself to overcome the restlessness that dispatches my mind on desperate tangents. If I were at home and not in this prison bed, I'd be rushing round madly, doing menial tasks like the dishes and weeding.

I'd never known Genevieve X not to be meticulously groomed. Her immaculate clothing sense and carriage were immediately noticeable. Most of our female friends adhered to basic standards of personal hygiene and clean clothes, but Mrs X was positively ascendant. It must have been the way she knotted a scarf round her shoulder or the soft colours she chose for her jumpers. Olive always said it's easier if you're as graceful as a swan to start with, but an additional element wove its magic.

One discordant note intruded into all that elegance. That such a laugh should issue forth from that stylish throat . . . it was halfway between a caw and a cackle. In happier times, her husband dubbed it her 'cawkle.' She'd no idea, and we didn't let on. She'd have been mortified beyond measure. Mrs X's cawkle was truly hideous to hear, but it meant she was ineffably happy.

Observing Genevieve X join us sartorially ordinary mortals as her husband's disease progressed was an experience I wished never to repeat. It signified deep depression. She tended her husband round the clock with nary a pause or a bleat. I think I've noted elsewhere the importance of medical spouses; allow me to say again that without a first-class one, a doctor is doomed to life in the second tier. Mrs X was the top of the top drawer. Now, she ensured that her husband's bodily indignities were cleaned up as soon as they happened. It had come to this.

'How is he today?' I knew the answer but wanted her response.

'Not any better, I'm afraid, but we're trying.' He was worse. She couldn't acknowledge it. I respected such spouses, determined to stave off the inevitable with intense effort. If only willing it could make it so.

'And you, Genevieve? You must look after yourself as well.' I knew she'd ignore this advice.

'Time for that . . . later,' she whispered.

'You'll be no good to your husband exhausted and –'

She cut me off, and rightly so. I said what I had to say and she did what she had to do.

'I can't do otherwise, Dexter, and please don't add any more pressure.' She was at breaking point. I knew it. She knew it. Worst of all, Dr X knew it.

'Rrrr.' Dr X contorted his chin. He could use his hands, barely. They'd contracted into claws.

'I think he needs to talk to me alone for a moment, Genevieve.'

She folded her arms, hands under her armpits, all the desolation of her heart leaking silently from her eyes as she stumbled out, head bent.

I sat on the edge of the bed. Dr X's weakness for bold stripes was well known. His surgery decor and ties bore testament to this love, which his wife refused to let prevail in the communal spaces of their home. Now his wasted frame rested on the boldest sheets imaginable, magenta and orange and lime-green bars, which contrasted nicely with the cedar four-poster bed. This evidence of spousal devotion caught at my throat.

'Dr –' throat clearing – 'X,' I said. 'We both know what it's come to.'

Outside the door, I heard a small sob.

The agitated man sank back into his pillow. His chin relaxed. Sublime relief flooded his features. He flung a hand at my black bag.

I didn't hesitate. 'Dr X, I think I'd better write out another prescription for your tablets. You'll have it here if you need it. Only get it filled if necessary.' I added the usual admonitions. In general, it was better for them to have something in hand, a security blanket, not a trophy. Some of my colleagues like Thucydides Hare might disagree. 'In the meantime, here's something to see you through. I'll leave them here, right by the bed, where you can reach them.'

Early next morning, the phone rang. I darted out a hand turtle-like and patted round the bedside table until cold instrument met warm flesh. My expression conveyed the worst to my wife. '. . . peacefully in his sleep during the night,' Mrs X sobbed.

I uttered I recall not what soothing words and burrowed my head into my dear wife's welcoming breast. 'Our turn will come,' she whispered. 'None of us knows what's round the corner.' We clung together as our years accordioned out and in, first endless then a matter of mere moments, two people toeing the abyss.

'May it be far away,' I murmured fervently into her soft centre.

It wasn't. It has arrived with breathtaking rapidity and ugliness. The facts sound so bald: Dr X suffered from multiple sclerosis contracted late in life. Eventually, he committed suicide by very, very nicely accumulating the tablets I'd given him and taking the whole lot at once. That's the truth of the matter. Brianna Bugden the femocrat got me for assisting a suicide by overprescribing. I either knew what I was doing or was incompetent. Did I wish to be remembered as criminally negligent?

This is what it's come to, all the years of leaving my warm wife's side willingly in the dead of night, my crazy schedule contorting family events, and round-the-clock service for patients who were never far from my heart. And still aren't. Now I've got the family to consider. I don't want this to come to trial again. One public spectacle is enough. Sometimes I wished we'd stayed in Britain.

Snakebite!

David Snow

One can know patients too well and miss signals. I tuned out Tom Allen's complaints about his wife for years. Big mistake. I should have been prepared, because it led to a chain of events culminating in a near-disaster.

Out here, we rely on our own skills and each other's. Our local nurses are generally quite competent, like Veronica Allen, but the ones the agency sends to remote areas can be crazy. Oddballs, like the Dutch nurse. She bewildered the permanent staff. To be honest, I felt the xenophobia common to small, isolated communities. That's part of it, but not all. Very abrupt she was, and eccentric as anything. It was she who was on duty the weekend a tiger snake bit Tom Allen.

The call came one Saturday afternoon at 3:00 from the State Emergency Service (SES). Mr Allen trod on a tiger snake when he and Mrs Allen were hiking way down the river track.

'Bring him in!' I said. 'Immediately!'

'It'll take us some hours, doc, but we'll be in as soon as we can,' said SES.

I did my hospital rounds about 7:00 that evening, a bit abstracted. Unfortunate the snake chose Tom Allen of all people. He was the most resentful person I'd ever met; aside from his wife, who kept hers hidden, something of which the poor man was incapable, to the discomfort of us all. Veronica gave up long ago importuning her husband to share her love of bushwalking. She'd only recently resumed the attack, with my encouragement. As a young married man, doctors misdiagnosed his porphyria as schizophrenia. He received shock treatments; not on my watch, thank God. My predecessor wore that one. After 19 months of ECT, an alert intern put two and two together and Tom was hastily released from further torture. I'd probably come out with a chip on my shoulder, too, and brain damage.

Meanwhile, Veronica returned to nursing to support three children under the age of five and a husband in and out of institutions. She bit the bullet and swallowed the rest. Her love of bushwalking parked itself on the mantelpiece in the living room, along with the first rosy blush of married life.

Out here, we're closer than most to Mother Nature. We humans are always yearning to merge. We go skiing, sailing, camping or bushwalking. We heed admonitions about loose snow or sharks or bears or snakes. Perhaps we spied a slash of something threatening and shivered in momentary watchfulness until the web of everyday woes redescended. Sister Allen knew all about that.

Tom's ECT left him with the shrillest voice I've ever heard in a man, part monotone and part shriek. It would dominate any marital dispute. As Tom couldn't hold down a job, my predecessor helped him obtain a disability pension. He had enough insight to know something was wrong and cover it up. He blamed his wife for urging him to go for treatment. I suspected his discontent about being a househusband, staying home and caring for the children. I monitored him discreetly when he brought them in for the usual childhood illnesses and accidents.

Tom splashed around like a child in a bathtub, hitting the waters of life with flat palms in his coping wars with daily reality. Veronica covered for him as time passed, except in the one area they chose as a battlefield: food. In this arena, each resentment festering in their hearts found voice. Tom did all the cooking, which he spiced with bitterness. His wife rejected his efforts. She insisted they were hazardous to the health. Tom's culinary disasters began as a joke at the nurses' station and ended in legend, simmering on the back burner alongside the other scabs and bruises of the Allen marriage. He was proud not to follow recipes. It didn't bother him if an ingredient was missing or unattractive. He just left it out. I tasted one of the rock cakes Veronica threw at the wall. She was right.

The years passed. The Allen brood sprouted, blossomed and departed. I'd observed the marital sniping slowly coming to the boil, but nothing more virulent than in other couples for whom time rubbed off the veneer of unmet expectations and blended them in the food processor of marriage. It was more of the same when Tom came in for his flu needle or brought one of the children. His damaged brain could not process his wife's preference for takeaway Chinese.

Two weeks before the snakebite, I was writing up some notes at the nursing station. Sister Allen belittled her husband's latest culinary creation. Those within earshot hooted their support, all except the Dutch nurse, who remained silent. I hated for Veronica's sharp edges to harden into habits while her softer side withered.

'We've been married 23 years now, and not once has he cooked a meal I've enjoyed. I'm not that fussy, but he doesn't have the knack, and he won't listen to me. He's got his way of doing things, and that's that.'

Veronica told me that Tom was unable or unwilling to learn new skills or update existing ones. I reiterated that brain damage from all those shock treatments may have been the cause. She told me he resisted computer lessons like he rejected woks and stir-fry, which she loved. He wasn't able to change his culinary repertoire. Veronica said eating his meals was like going into a time warp. 'If it was good enough for me mum and dad, it's good enough for Her,' he shrieked in that awful voice of his.

'Why don't you resume bushwalking?' I suggested. I don't know where that came from, but fortunately my diagnostic skills hadn't completely deserted me. 'You loved it so.'

She laughed. 'You know Tom, doctor. Can you imagine our picnic lunch . . .'

'Give it a go. Might be the best thing for both of you.' She needed to do something, anything, to keep from sliding into that yawning abyss of peppery needles that swallowed so many couples.

She patted her hips. 'You're right. They have spread.'

'Don't get hurt,' said the Dutch nurse disapprovingly. 'We're short-staffed. As usual. And you, doctor,' she rounded on me. 'Don't ask me to do anything else. I'm too busy. Do a few things yourself around here.'

We all looked forward to the end of school holidays and the expiration of her locum.

The emergency service brought Tom in at 9:00 that evening. Most people who are bitten by snakes are not envenomated. It'll bite, but not inject the venom, so the doctor simply monitors the patient overnight to watch for any reaction. Tom was unlucky. His eyes were already dilated when I saw him. Poison paralyses the eye muscles, so his vision was blurred and he'd already been vomiting for a number of hours.

I knew he felt terrible because he'd curled up into the foetal position, but I asked anyway, 'How do you feel, mate?'

'Like death warmed up. It's all her fault. I never wanted to go.' Blaming the wife became a way of life.

Venom paralyses the nervous system and stops the blood from clotting, so we took a test sample from Tom. It didn't clot. We took more blood later with the same result. He was significantly envenomated and could die in 24 hours.

'Right, we'll treat Mr Allen,' I said to the room.

We needed two things: antivenom, which came from horses, and good advice, which came from the public hospital down in our capital, hundreds of miles away. Of our two lots of antivenom, one was slightly out of date. I told the Dutch nurse that we needed more and she should ring the hospital in the next town.

'This may be enough. Let's try it and see.'

'I said we need more. Get on the phone now!'

'No!'

'We haven't got time for this!' I'd report this bitch as soon as things calmed down.

'I'll do it,' said the cleaner, whose sister-in-law was the charge nurse at the closer hospital. As to our second need, often in remote areas it's hard to find good advice. A lot of 'experts' don't know what they're talking about. I hadn't treated snakebite in all my 15 years, and wanted to discuss a few things. Sister Allen did all the right first aid, swathed his whole arm in a bandage. Despite that, he was still envenomated. I wanted to know if you remove the bandage before you give the antivenom or give the antivenom and remove the bandage, in case additional poison is released into the system. I also needed to find out how much antivenom to give. I rang up the city hospital. It was one of their busy times, approaching 12:00 on a Saturday night.

'Gimme your accident and emergency department.'

They put me through.

'Right, give me your most senior person on call.'

'That's Dr Mubbly-Bubbly-Mumbly.' They gave a name that was 2 metres long, and a subcontinental accent came on the line.

'Hello, yes?'

'Have you ever treated a tiger snake bite?'

If he'd said no, I'd have said, 'Thank you very much, I need to speak to somebody else.' But he said instead, 'What have you got?'

'A guy who's been bitten by a tiger snake and envenomated. How much antivenom do I give him? I have 2 units.'

'Well, you give a little bit, and then a little bit more.'

'Right. Thank you very much, that's been very helpful,' I said, and put the phone down. I rang back and asked, 'Who's in charge of ICU tonight?'

'Dr B, but we can't find him. We tried earlier.'

'Can you page Dr Van Deutsch?' We were classmates at university, and now he was director of accident and emergency. They put me through. After the preliminaries, I asked, 'Have you ever treated a tiger snake bite, Deutschy?'

'Yes, two.'

'Fine, how much antivenom do you give?'

'The standard dose is 2 units, but you'll probably have to give more if he's been properly envenomated.'

'And the bandage?'

'That doesn't matter. You can take it off because he's been envenomated. It's pointless now.'

'Righto. How do you monitor how much antivenom you have to give?'

'By the clotting in the blood. As soon as you get the prothrombin ratio back down to near normal, you know you've given enough antivenom.'

I knew the effects were not immediate. Taking the blood in half an hour would give me time to round up the pathologist. The Dutch nurse and I were at Tom's bedside when the cleaner approached. 'Excuse me, doctor,' she said. 'My sister-in-law is in one of her difficult moods. You'd better talk to her.'

'Carry on here,' I said to the Dutch nurse as I ran into the corridor. 'I'll be back as soon as I can.'

'No,' she said. 'I don't think I will. What I think is –'

'It's not your job to think! Just do it!'

She turned to the patient, thank God, disapproval oozing from every pore.

I grabbed the phone at the nurse's station. 'Yes . . . yes . . . the thing is, we only have 2 units of antivenom, and one is out of date . . . No . . .' I imagined ringing all round the district. It was now midnight. 'Look,' I said, 'I know you don't want to part with yours in case you need it, but it's fairly unlikely at midnight you're going to get a case of snakebite. We need to treat something which has already happened. Send me the bloody antivenom.'

We'd already alerted the police and the cops brought it over.

So we treated Mr Allen. His initial prothrombin ratio was not recordable because the blood didn't clot. When you treat someone with warfarin to lower it, normal is 2–3 INR. When we got his prothrombin ratio down to 2.5, I said, 'Right, that's enough, we can all go home.'

Next day, I did my rounds after church. 'How do you feel now, mate?' I asked Tom.

'Better. I'm never letting her talk me into anything. It's all her fault.'

I rang up Hobart and got Van Deutsch. 'What do we do now?'

'Is he feeling better?'

'Yeah, significantly.'

'He can go home.'

Mr Allen subsequently suffered all the problems associated with tissue breakdown. It overloaded his kidneys, so we sent him for dialysis for a number of weeks, but he recovered.

We got rid of the Dutch nurse.

Veronica Allen formed a bushwalking group. No one minded that her husband refused to join. Tom supports his wife's hobby by making food he lovingly dehydrates, which she scatters to the winds.

The virgin and the ▬ roadster

Malcolm Phillips

> Some people call you out for every whiffle of a sniffle: 'You've got to come and give me antibiotics.' Why should I have to go out to them when they're perfectly capable of going out shopping and to the races? Why can't they come to the surgery? When I suggest this, they whinge and carry on. All I can say is, thank God for government participation in medical practice.

Don't be misled by frequent grumbling. Not all doctors perceive the third party as the enemy. It's unequivocally the doctor's best friend. Ignore the discontent of a few paranoid colleagues. Yes, there's more paperwork for the same pay, but on the other hand we are now paid for what was formerly done as charity. The reality of modern medicine is usually a fruitful and happy partnership between patients, doctors and the third party: government and or/private insurer who pays for their consultations.

I was one of the first to computerise. I read somewhere that in Australia the percentage of GPs with computers on their desks increased from 15% in 1998 to 91% in 2005.[11] Patients have to move with the times. If it bothers them that I now spend part of my consultation time inputting their data instead of eyeballing them, they can go elsewhere. I can't be expected to spend hours on data entry at the end of a long day. And I have access to hard science on which to base my decisions. Evidence-based medicine, that's for me. Prescribing is so much easier with the computer. Some of them squawk about privacy and confidentiality, but adequate controls are in place. Some colleagues fret that time spent tapping a keyboard during consultations may allow important cues to be missed, but I haven't found this to be the case.

Perhaps the softer patients have gone elsewhere, along with the mobile ones. That's fine with me. I never liked wimps of either sex, or battlers for that matter. Let them go to the bleeding hearts. I'll have mine full of beans, and preferably speaking the same language, like two emotionally robust patients: BOBs, my wife calls them. Bitter old bags. Acerbic elderly femininity, a welcome antidote to all

11 Pearce and Trumble 2006.

that earnest sweetness. My son once said Miss Citroen looked as if she'd been sucking lemons. I called her the Virgin Queen and my other BOB the Roadster. Miss Amelia Carlyle had been round the block a few times.

Miss Faith Citroen was a different sort of war casualty, but walking wounded nonetheless. She didn't march in parades or haunt graves clutching flowers, tears rolling down her cheeks. Hers was a grand passion of the sort that only coalesces once in a lifetime. BOB Number One spent a life pining for love lost. The Second World War threw her off balance. Lucky in birth, unlucky in love. The whole town knew that hers was far from the tragic romance she pretended. Yes, she'd lost her fiancé in the war, but not through death. He'd met someone else over there, brought her back and lived happily ever after in a city not 2 hours' drive away. Word got round, as these things do. Everyone knew the truth or an embroidered version, allowing the spinster to save face in that sublime way of villages.

The act of regaining equilibrium manifested in constant motion, going from event to event, race to show. One wondered what she was running from in her efforts to 'keep amused', as she drawled, jabbing the air with her cane. Arthritis stooped her tall frame, but did not soften her angularity, physical and otherwise. Nor did the love of a pet – an emotion she reciprocated with all the fierceness of her nature. Her Jack Russell terrier barked incessantly in a high-pitched frenzy that made me want to kick it. Later, when she died, her family asked the vet to put it down. Just as well. They were a twosome no one else could love.

Miss Citroen's heart turned to stone over time, and her body followed. Ossification was almost complete when I inherited her. Her tombstone was in sight. She got about with a cane, but haltingly, so I usually saw her at home. Some said she was a snob, but her vitality-sucking negativity didn't affect me. Indeed, it was a relief to call on a patient closer to my own social situation.

One evening at dusk, I turned off the road into Miss Faith's drive. The oceanic expanse of fine white pebbles replacing green lawn left me gasping in wonderment. She'd done it in the late 1940s and must have refreshed it regularly for the pebbles to sparkle so. In the exact middle arose a crumbling stone sundial. The juxtaposition of ultramodern and antique worked a charm. No other ornament or shrub diluted the effect of this Zen garden. The local rumour mill insisted she'd done it not for purposes of contemplation but practicality. This was to have been her starter home with her betrothed. She planned to travel. She wasn't a stay-at-home, gardening type, she informed him. This modest house was meant to be a temporary perch on her upward trajectory. After the war, she ripped out every living thing that grew in front of the house and suffocated the fertile ground. The process of petrifaction had begun.

I alighted from the car and pulled my truffle-coloured cashmere muffler close, appreciating its gentle warmth. The coral sky heralded a frosty morning. I approached La Citroen's house, painted cream with green trim, and tugged the bell pull near the front door. I preferred it to the knocker. No rustling response sounded within. 'Dr Phillips,' I called out. As my patient was elderly, I eased open the door and started down the passageway, over the Turkey carpet that levelled the uneven flagstones. I entered the lounge.

A stench assaulted my olfactory sense: the room reeked of urine. This was where the house's inhabitant spent most of her time. A quick survey of the dimly lit room revealed it to be empty of human presence. I surveyed the *mémentos de guerre* while deciding whether to go upstairs or sing out. Photographs of châtelaine and horses, equine awards and race-meeting invitations displayed the detritus of a life lived alone. The room's dissonance disturbed me. An oddly uninhabited feeling permeated the room, as if its owner merely perched between outings. All the right *things* were in place – a veritable stage set – but instead of amusing their owner, they thrust her farther afield. No computer, television or music system spoke of the modern age. My surroundings were frozen in time. Life had stopped 70 years ago. The trauma of lost love trapped one heart forevermore.

A demure cough raised me from my reveries. A figure rose from the shadows of an armchair. I experienced that jolt one does upon realising one is not alone in a room.

That Miss Citroen was a survivor shone in her forward limping gait – like a headstrong sheep which brooks no opposition – and in the determined cast of her mouth. Her eyes said something else.

'Not exactly the flagged and panelled interior I grew up with.' She waved an insouciant hand at the room and passageway. 'Good of you to come, doctor.' Her tone told me I was a tolerated but necessary intruder. 'Help yourself to sherry.'

'Thank you, think I will.' I strode to the drinks trolley, selected a glass and decanted the golden liquid from its crystal home.

'I've got nuts somewhere.' She flapped her hand dismissively. Her manner conveyed her feelings. I brushed aside my reaction, which did not belong in the repertoire of a healer. Pain affected people. This woman found none of my predecessors worthy, but they wielded the magic prescription pad. I joined a long line of inepts, the *not quite quites*.

A worn airline packet of peanuts was gathering dust on an occasional table. 'No, thanks,' I said, glancing at a photograph of her younger days, all hat and attitude.

'That's me at Ascot. I'd gone over to, well, it doesn't concern you.' She adjusted the lacy collar on a grey silk dress, wispy as her hair, which fashion left behind generations ago. I suspected she'd worn it in the first blush of youth between the wars. By the onset of the Second World War, Miss Citroen's attire would have been considered quaint indeed. Now, one felt a participant in a period piece: Noel Coward with Prim Unpleasant Aunt.

I strode past a chair placed over a hole in the Chinese carpet and sank into peach-coloured down cushions upon which peacocks cavorted, appreciating the sofa's quality.

'Next to you on the little inlaid table is a photograph taken before my back gave out.'

I gazed at a younger image of my patient at a Hunt Club do. 'Is that why you've called me out?'

'Yes, doctor, the pain. Must be the change of weather . . .'

She seemed no worse than usual, but one cannot always tell with people who habitually hide their feelings.

'Give me more of those tablets.' She fingered her collar. 'I'm going to the races tomorrow and I'm driving. You know Mrs Tunbridge. She's invited Carlyle, that dreadful social climber. Mrs Tunbridge is a bit muddled – that's nothing new – she'd never have done such a thing in the old days. She always got by on her looks. By the time they faded, she'd hooked Mr Tunbridge. I always said he could have done better.' Her complexion suffused with malicious pleasure. 'There aren't many of us left, and our kind have to stick together.'

'Yes that's exactly right.'

She snorted. 'I wasn't thinking of you, far from it. At any rate, it's convenient for you to come to me. You can't stare into a computer the whole time.'

I smiled with impish delight and pulled out a Blackberry. I'd got the upper hand.

My patient raised her eyebrows to her hairline and looked at me down the bridge of her nose, ensuring that I knew I was no more to her than Howard the mechanic. He fixed her car; I kept her body on the road. She respected me less because she couldn't worm out of paying him.

Part of me felt contemptuous that she'd not the social equipment to recognise a 'younger son' when she saw one. Another part lashed out like a wounded boy desperate for acceptance.

The sherry tasted rough. The spinster's acid seeped into the amber liquid, corroding another relationship. It was pure romantic nonsense, my quip about a heart trapped forevermore. She was born to belittle, which her betrothed comprehended just in time.

I scribbled a prescription that enabled her life of constant motion. She'd too many miles on the odometer to attempt a detour. Miss Faith Citroen barely glanced at the Medicare form she signed. She wasn't a charity case, but that was the only way I'd be paid for that consultation.

Yes, government participation is the doctor's best friend.

The third party can provide a different sort of refuge. Patients sometimes demolish one, despite the encrusting armour that comes with time. Lemony BOB and BOB Number Two exemplified two types of aloneness and spinsterhood, too good for everybody and good enough for everyone. I craved acceptance from Miss Faith Citroen. Considering her to be a caricature took the edge off her rejection. For all her constant motion, she never travelled widely enough – defined as overseas – to recognise herself as a big fish in a little pond. She lorded – ladied – it over other unsophisticates, who themselves preferred the comforts of home to international exploration. Buying into the same game gave it power. Miss Faith Citroen sailed along full of misconceptions regarding my own birth, of which I did not disabuse her. My relatives would laugh at her – in private, of course.

Miss Amelia Carlyle the Roadster came from across the water. This gave her a broader view of life than that of her arrogant friend. A few women were well known by all the men in the district and fondly remembered for freely distributing their favours. Eileen the shearers' cook was one. Miss Amelia was another, an ex-publican with a loose reputation and a well-born mother. The latter caused the Roadster no end of grief and yearning in our class-ridden town. Miss Citroen ignored her until most of their generation died off. The Roadster always trotted out – fruitlessly – her exalted mother from landed gentry on the mainland. Miss Faith occasionally allowed BOB Number Two to accompany her to the races, especially as she was mobile and able to drive, and comfortably off enough to replace her car every 2 years.

The Roadster called me out one late afternoon in sweltering midsummer. My linen jacket kept me cool. As it was wrinkled, I'd have to exchange it for a fresher one before tonight's do at the club. I'd been asked to give a speech. I reviewed it as I negotiated the weed-cracked crazy paving, past a stunted camellia, round to the back of a stucco-and-stone house the colour of an old crankshaft.

Another garden taught me what my patient wished not to reveal. While her friend's wedge of earth was all cold white Zen pebbles with a tiny back patch dominated by clothesline leading to massive rolling paddocks, Miss Amelia Carlyle kept her front anonymous, reminiscent of those Middle Eastern and American Southern homes with great walls backing onto the street and flowering into a fairyland within. Her backyard was tropical in its lush viridescence, dominated by potato vines and clematis crawling from three ancient lilac trees to a bank of green-black shrubs.

The ex-publican sat in a cane armchair on the veranda nursing a gin and tonic. 'Come and sit down, doctor,' she said. She was small and round, with large brown eyes, finely sculpted nose and hands and the peaches-and-cream complexion of someone who spent little time out of doors. 'Help yourself to a drink.' She flapped her hand as had the Virgin Queen at a drinks trolley nearby.

I poured a small sherry and joined her at the table. The first Norah Jones CD played in the background.

Miss Amelia looked off-colour, possibly reflected from all that verdure. She'd lived a lifetime among the urgent needs of men, something the Roadster knew well, having been the main comfort of all the better-bred males in the district. People's memories sheltered a lot of history. When the fabric tore, she restitched it with embroidered truth. She was overly generous to men – except her nephew, whom she despised – and was always offering us food. Another side of patients' gifts is bribery, perhaps unconscious. They proffer such items as teddy bears, chocolate biscuits and old coins. The 85-year-old Roadster genuinely liked people. Unfortunately, the juice that drove her engine mixed itself with vitriol. Miss Faith's was the only presence which subdued her.

The addition of the fruits of her own business acumen combined with discreet legacies from wistful old gents made the ex-publican quite comfortably off, more so than Miss Faith, which they both knew and exploited. Their traits intensified as they grew older. Miss Faith became a caricature of snobbishness. Miss Amelia bifurcated, treating women abysmally – except for Miss Faith – and men of all ages with great tenderness, excluding her sister's boy, who lived down the street in one of her run-down houses. He felt the full force of her tongue. As a doctor, I occupied uncensored emotional territory.

'Mrs S across the way wants to come with us to the races but I refuse to invite her. Faith wouldn't approve.' She leaned forward confidentially. 'You know of course that Faith's lamented fiancé is happily married down in the capital. Has been since the war.'

A metallic glint from the lounge room caught my eye. I peered into a room conspicuously devoid of photographs. A sole painting hung over the mantel in the lounge room, in pride of place: a portrait of the queen and a rather ducal, familiar-looking character that my hostess claimed as an ancestor. Copper kettles of all sizes and shapes squatted on the mantelpiece like little soldiers, lean and ruddy. Roped to one was a blue-and-white delft china handle.

'. . . Faith doesn't know men like I do,' she was saying.

I nodded.

'And another thing, doctor. Just because Mrs S married a retired doctor, that doesn't confer the legitimacy she thinks it does. Prefers older men, does she? Plenty of decrepit shearers and demented farmhands in the old folks' home, I told her. She ignored me. Dr S only married her to avoid paying for a round-the-clock housekeeper and nurse. I expect she'll do well enough out of it, especially as she's got a sharp lawyer. She can buy all the designer clothes she wants but she can't hide that huge bum of hers. What a waddle! It's deportment that tells. And the way she looks at my nephew, that good-for-nothing, as if she's lining up her next victim. He responds – men always do, you know – so I've changed my will. Won't she be surprised! Won't he! Hope she marries him before I'm cold. I'm leaving it all to the church. The sisters brought me up after Mother died. They were admirable. But I'm not disinheriting poor Jason entirely. I'm leaving him the house he's living in.'

'But that needs quite a lot of work, doesn't it?'

'Yes,' she said with a wicked glint and small smile.

I changed the subject. 'You're playing my favourite Norah Jones CD.'

'Christmas present from my nephew. I'm surprised at your lack of musical sophistication, doctor. Now Sheryl Crow is something else entirely, as I'm always telling that lazy good-for-nothing.' She closed her eyes, breathing harder.

'What's the trouble today, Miss Carlyle?'

'Amelia, please, as I keep telling you, doctor.' She added, bestowing a benediction, 'My friends call me Mel.'

I said nothing, but watched my patient.

'I made some soup yesterday, my lovely home-made pumpkin soup, on the bench top in the old margarine tub. Please have it, doctor.' She twirled her gin and tonic.

'No, thank you. Tell me what's happened.'

'I'd a dizzy turn last night, and with my eyes I felt it was better not to go out.'

'You've done the right thing, Miss – Amelia. Mel.'

'Jason is useless. He doesn't have a car, and I'm not giving him mine.'

'Let's see what we can find.' I felt in my bag for the sphygmomanometer. 'I can't take a history if you're on the G&T.'

Miss Amelia replaced her glass painstakingly in the centre of a tiny round cane table. Her hand refused to obey properly. I'd never have observed this in the surgery. She flailed without her liquid prop. 'I'm a little shaky, doctor, since Mr Strait died last week. I'd known him for 45 years. He was one of the loves of my life. Saved him from an embarrassing and expensive mistake with Ms Tiffany. His wife didn't appreciate what I did for her. And Faith's brother, and her father: I knew them as well as she did.'

'I'm sure the women round here owe you a great debt.'

'You'd be surprised,' she said, eyes softening as she dipped into her memories. 'We're almost like family, you know.'

I couldn't destroy an old lady's illusions. 'I'm going to call an ambulance to take you to town. You need a going-over. Why are you frowning?'

'I'm trying to decide if you should know what my friend truly thinks of you.' She knew how to manipulate men, how to spot weakness and control the beast.

'Miss Citroen is getting on, and pain does funny things,' I said, sensing trouble.

'Some things never change. She's always called you "the monkey", you know: a climber. Not really one of us. Not from the top drawer. I told her that you were a "younger son", but she just laughed.'

'Best to prepare for several days away,' I said, a little too severely.

'Just thought you should know,' she said sweetly.

That was last week. I'm tired of going out at all hours to demanding old ladies and am considering a new profession in the pharmaceutical industry. Drug companies know how to enhance one's *amour propre*.

There's a postscript to this story. Fate deposited Miss Amelia and Miss Citroen in the same nursing home. By this time, their relationship had deteriorated into uncompromising honesty. Staff housed them in different wings and had strict instructions to keep them separated at all times, no mean feat in these days of increasingly motorised wheelchairs and diminishing hereditary entitlement.

Sued

Dexter Veriform

'The time has come, Olive Oil. Please,' I pleaded, waving my bandaged forearms at my wife of 52 years, mother of our four children. 'Please don't fail me or foil me. Remember what we promised each other. No lingering indignities.' I shifted in my bed, as if shackles would allow me to get closer to my beloved wife. We're one being now, and have been throughout living memory. No cataclysmic event heralded the fusion. I simply looked at her across the toast one morning, she glanced up, read my mind and that was that. Now, eyes streaming, she stares down at me on the prison hospital bed. She knows what I want, and baulks. I know, and despair.

Aside from the obvious deprivations of prison life, I miss my animals. I miss the smell of dog breath, the feel of a healthy coat and the joyous welcoming bark. I long for that special love animals radiate. I remember Otis, the Border collie Mr Stevens left me. The poor man lost his lovely wife and contracted a nasty carcinoma of the bowel. He was the one who shot himself neatly by the incinerator. Otis languished after that. One of my farmer friends suggested that it might be kindest to shoot him – nice symmetry, that. Alas, it was not within my capabilities. Nor was fobbing off that responsibility onto the veterinarian. Otis failed to thrive and soon joined Mr Stevens. I saw that so much in people as well: suddenly, they'd no reason to hang around. Now our tenuous hold on existence is brought home to me, that tissue-thin veil so easily pierced. I feel it parting.

The femocrat accuses me of murdering Dr X. What really bothers me is the way she bandies about 'betrayal of trust.' Never! Never never *never*. My God, it has underpinned my entire professional life. What would *she* know? Who's begged her to put a shotgun to their heads, same as they'd do for the dog? Which of her beloved flock has she watched deteriorating inexorably, despite the fiercest determination of all concerned? What children has she watched sacrifice their fleeting childhoods, year after year, to tend a brain-damaged incontinent vegetative sibling? How . . . dare . . . she . . .

Betrayal of trust. Have I lived too long? Yes I'm practising medicine well into my 70s; at least, I was until the present debacle. I couldn't let my old patients down. We grew old together and needed each other. They begged me not to retire, some in so many words, others with signals, jokes and allusions. Life was unimaginable without them. My work was my life. I didn't mind being called out at night or at weekends. Even if the reason seemed trivial or was buried beneath their comprehension. Now I can't go anywhere. Prison! My God! I always did the things that mattered. I never kept my patients waiting for a minute longer than necessary. The representatives of pharmaceutical companies knew I wouldn't see them until I'd attended to all the session's patients and emergencies. I always gave my patients scripts if they wanted, sometimes with the admonition not to get them filled unless it was necessary. I tried to empower them, to educate them about their illnesses if they were so inclined and to give them plenty of time. I was no autocrat like Thucydides Hare.

Am I such an anachronism? Didn't I do enough? I followed the golden rule, and was I ever done unto in the end! I was too busy to take in medical students and trainees. My honest patients were disconcerted by the presence of a third person. I refused to put them in the position of having to be polite. One on one. That's how it should be. Anything else upsets the balance of power and personal interaction. I'd have hated it if a patient, who finally worked up the nerve to reveal a problem with the waterworks that had bothered him for years, was deterred by the presence of a determined young female student who only intended to work as a lifestyle consultant 1 day a week to preserve her quality of life. Or an earnest male the age of his grandson. Let them learn another way.

And something else. I faced them instead of tapping away at a computer keyboard. What I want to know is often found in the way they say it, not the words they utter. In the end, it wasn't a patient's signal that I missed. I was forced out by something sinister gnawing at the very core of our calling.

Somewhere along the line, the gem was lost and we don't know how to retrieve it. Lord save me from the watchdogs, from transparency, accountability and regulation. I'm a healer. I'm accountable to a higher source, and that's all I'll answer to. I agree with Raymond Tallis. In a suspicious, over-regulated society, moral cowardice can rule decision-making.[12] Everybody's morally petrified into inaction. I'm proud to say I never let it happen to me. We have no protectors, especially if we don't play the game. Don't start squawking at me. I know all about doctors' protection organisations. Fat lot of good they did me.

It saddens me that I will never again gaze out my study window at the silvereye alighting on the dogwoods, *Cornus alba* 'Sibirica', whose winter stems glow such a glossy crimson. They're so unassuming the rest of the year, with their rounded leaves and tiny clusters of white flowers, but they shine when other plants hibernate. Their leaves burnish, brown and crackle with the passing months, fading to chartreuse or transparent rose. Silvereyes and Siberian dogwoods belong to a receding world.

My patients are hovering round my bed. Here's Sandy MacSalter in Scotland, the poor brain-damaged boy I didn't treat when he contracted meningitis. His death was a great relief to his family. Hello, Wee Donnie MacKay. Remember that time you wielded your gun? I prevented a mass murder and facilitated a marriage. I treated your cousin Maggie Reid as a teenager with multiple sclerosis, and we're in touch after all these years. Here's Wiley Riley from New Zealand, with his prize-winning bull and his miscarrying wife. He nearly lost that pregnant filly – would have if I'd not followed my intuition. It's always come through for

---

12 Tallis 2004. p. 105.

me. Hello Ewan Graymouth, with your Christmas goose, and the Jack family with *il trombe ultimo*. And poor old Iris McBride, she of the sedate Sunday morning drive to church. Whoople the Cadger has won.

Another patient floats by, unbelievably scruffy, with creased trousers, an open-necked shirt, a button off here and day-old stubble on the jaw. What was his name? Can't recall. My memory's fading. Heart of gold. I never left his farm without eggs or spuds, nor can I recall ever buying them in New Zealand. One of the odd side effects of the health service was that, because patients weren't required to pay, you'd receive a little gift if they felt pleased with you. That was before the Entitlement Generation. I got all sorts of things. One alcoholic patient gave me a television set that didn't work terribly well.

Olive liked to watch Dr Finlay on the telly. He didn't know how lucky he was, being able to devote himself to his practice, with Annette Crosbie as his housekeeper, Janet, and no wife or children. Was ever doctor more devoted to patient? The good man came to fisticuffs with one, a Charlie Bell with 'small, derisive eyes, and a close-cropped, brick-red head.'[13] He told another she was a terrible mother who didn't love her child when he was 'stung beyond endurance by her icy indifference' to her boy's suffering.[14]

If I have one plea to you, it's to give medicine back to the doctors. Wrest it from the bureaucrats, and we'll begin to reattract healers and not business people and part-timers to the profession. Abolish immediately all paperwork required aside from note-taking, letters to specialists, medical reports and other scribblings arising from clinical practice. Does the rest of it really matter? Let the bureaucrats go off and plague some other profession for a while. Why have we handed over health and well-being? Claim them back! For God's sake, do it now or only pen-pushers and materialists will populate our profession.

'Oh, hello, doctor. We showed that femocrat at the conference for continuing-education points, didn't we? Patients it is to the end, not clients. Good of you to come.' Here was just the person I needed to see. 'I wasn't sure Olive conveyed the message. I need your help on a little matter. Olive's lost heart. Can't say I blame her. I know she'll understand, at least I hope so. Thank you doctor, leave them near my right hand.'

And thank God thank God thank God.

One of my favourite patients is beckoning. I'd forgotten Mrs Bliscott. I called her Snipper, a private nickname for a sweet lady of 89 years who made a snip-ping motion with the first two fingers of her right hand. She developed the tic in later years. I loved the old dear. She'd been feeling very unwell and finally rang me early one morning. Her speech was so slurred I barely understood her. I rang the ambulance straight away and got through to the night sister on the first attempt. By the time I arrived at hospital, the old dear was in a coma. I sat with her all through the early hours, holding her hand as she crossed the rainbow bridge. That's the term I use to small children to explain the endless desertion of pet birds and fish.

We communicated despite Mrs Bliscott's unconsciousness, until the end. I recalled our conversations over the years. She told me about growing up in the

13 Cronin 1969. p. 50.
14 Ibid. p. 93.

bush, and I told her about my childhood outside London. Her oldest sister was sacrificed at the age of twelve to a travelling salesman, who bought her for a sum of money and a flesh-pink, perfectly preserved antique Chinese silk shawl with 9 inches of fringe. I recalled the skirmishes and ambushes of four little boys on the battlefield of parental love. Her father followed sheep to shave them bald. Mine counted shepherds among his best friends but ignored his own sons. Her tired mother sent her brood out to exhaust themselves in the birch grove with leaves tinkling under the dappled afternoon sun. My dutiful *maman* sent her sons away to be birched by pedants. Mrs Bliscott remembered crunching over a coating of sycamore leaves that burred the autumn earth and browned the horizon. I recalled the fall of Father, a tree trunk silhouetted on a pockmarked moonscape. She embraced the love of men. I evaded the wiles of women. She gave scones fresh from the oven to hungry men. I presented my half-baked dreams, which times cooled and staled to hard little rock cakes. Mrs Bliscott cooked grilled sausages and mountains of spuds for her shearers. I spoke parings of wisdom, peppered with avalanches of facts and presented to numberless patients.

I wasn't able to pinpoint the exact moment of Mrs Bliscott's death. It was a process of gradual withdrawing, like the cooling down of an overheated engine. As I'm feeling now. I pray that my patients learned as much from me as they taught me. When I became a doctor, I never knew my patients would inspire me with awe. I felt more kinship with Snipper Bliscott than with most of my colleagues, certainly Thucydides Hare. I valued her counsel deeply. She's snipping at one end of the night rainbow. I'm nipping at the other. The massive bowl of night overflows with a milky froth.

Does that low wail belong to my Olive? '*Come back*' threads through the clouds across a crescent moon, like a last jar of home-made jam, the final offering from a grateful patient.

I hope I've given as much as I've received.

Bibliography

Animal Pictures Archive. Green-and-Black Streamertail Hummingbird (*Trochilus polytmus*). Available at: www.animalpicturesarchive.com/view.php?tid=3&did=26919 (accessed 19 November 2011).

Bailey H. *Hamilton Bailey's Demonstrations of Physical Signs in Clinical Surgery*, 15th ed. Bristol: John Wright & Sons; 1973.

Balzac H de. *The Fatal Skin*. New York: Signet; 1963.

Butler S. *Secrets from the Black Bag*. London: RCGP Publications; 2005.

Cairney S, Maruff P, Burns CB, *et al*. Saccade dysfunction associated with chronic petrol sniffing and lead encephalopathy. *J Neurol Neurosurg Psychiatry*. 2004; 75(3): 472–6.

Champion M. Aboriginal Religion and Christianity: fundamentally incompatible. 1995. Available at: www.ad2000.com.au/articles/1995/mar1995p10_848.html (accessed 18 November 2011).

Cronin AJ. *Adventures of a Black Bag*. London: New English Library; 1969.

Dalrymple T. *Romancing Opiates: pharmacological lies and the addiction bureaucracy*. New York: Encounter; 2006.

Emoto M. *The Secret Life of Water*. London: Simon and Schuster; 2005.

Fessler DMT, Pillsworth EG, Flamson TJ. Angry men and disgusted women: an evolutionary approach to the influence of emotions on risk taking. *Organ Behav Hum Decis Process*. 2004; 95: 107–23.

GlobalSecurity. *Diego Garcia 'Camp Justice' 7°20'S 72°25'E*. Available at: www.global security.org/military/facility/diego-garcia.htm (accessed 18 November 2011).

Gyatso T. When the gem was mine. *BODHI Times*. 1992; No 3, December.

Harcourt School Publishers. *An Eyewitness Account of the Eruption of Vesuvius*. Available at: www.harcourtschool.com/activity/pompeii/pmpMsStb.html (accessed 2 December 2011).

Helman C. *Suburban Shaman: tales from medicine's front line*. London: Hammersmith; 2006.

Lateef F, Anantharaman V. Maritime radio-medical services: the Singapore General Hospital experience. *Am J Emerg Med*. 2002; 20(4): 349–51.

Legislative Assembly of the Northern Territory. *Petrol Sniffing in Remote Northern Territory Communities*. Darwin: Select Committee on Substance Abuse in the Community; 2004.

Manson-Bahr PEC, Bell DR. *Manson's Tropical Diseases*. 19th ed. London: Ballière Tindall; 1987.

Ouspensky PD. *Strange Life of Ivan Osokin*. Baltimore, MD: Penguin; 1973.

Pearce C, Trumble S. Computers can't listen – algorhythmic logic meets patient centredness. *Aust Fam Physician*. 2006; 35(6): 439–42.

Pelisek C. Death of the snow cone man. *LA Weekly*. 2007 Jan 31. Available at: www. laweekly.com/2007-02-01/news/death-of-the-snow-cone-man (accessed 17 February 2012).

Sanger D, Feldman J. The conman, the dictator & the CIA files. *Daily Telegraph Magazine*. 20 June 1998. Available at: www.guardianlies.com/section%206/page35.html (accessed 19 November 2011).

Sava G. *The Healing Knife: a surgeon's destiny*. Harmondsworth: Penguin; 1953.

Soubiran A. *The Doctors*. Trans Oliver Coburn. London: WH Allen; 1954.

Soubiran A. *The Healing Oath*. Trans Oliver Coburn. London: WH Allen; 1954.

Stone DG. *'Monsters' of the Sea*. Available at: www.cryptozoology.com/articles/monstersofthesea.php (accessed 17 November 2011).

Tallis R. *Hippocratic Oaths*. London: Atlantic; 2004. p. 105.

Tsundue T. *Kora: stories and poems*. 4th ed. TibetWrites; 2007. Available at: www.tibetwrites.org/IMG/pdf/kora.pdf (accessed 17 February 2012).

Untermeyer L. The dog of Pompeii. In Allison C, editor. *Teach Your Children Well*. New York: Delacorte Press; 1993.

Willis J. *The Paradox of Progress*. Oxford: Radcliffe Medical Press; 1995.

World Resources Institute Archive. *Marine-Based Sources of Threat*. Available at: http://marine.wri.org/pubs_content_text.cfm?ContentID=3057 (accessed 19 November 2011).

Young W. Hidding and his brethren? *Tasmanian Times*. 16 March 2006. Available at: http://tasmaniantimes.com/index.php?/article/hidding-and-his-brethren (accessed 18 November 2011).